The New
Contented Little
Baby Book

Gina Ford

The New
Contented Little
Baby Book

The Secret to
Calm and Confident Parenting

NAL New American Library

New American Library
Published by the Penguin Group
Penguin Group (USA) Inc., 375 Hudson Street,
New York, New York 10014, USA
Penguin Group (Canada), 90 Eglinton Avenue East, Suite 700, Toronto,
Ontario M4P 2Y3, Canada (a division of Pearson Penguin Canada Inc.)
Penguin Books Ltd., 80 Strand, London WC2R 0RL, England
Penguin Ireland, 25 St. Stephen's Green, Dublin 2,
Ireland (a division of Penguin Books Ltd.)
Penguin Group (Australia), 707 Collins Street Melbourne, Victoria 3008,
Australia (a division of Pearson Australia Group Pty. Ltd.)
Penguin Books India Pvt. Ltd., 11 Community Centre, Panchsheel Park,
New Delhi–110 017, India
Penguin Group (NZ), 67 Apollo Drive, Rosedale, Auckland 0632,
New Zealand (a division of Pearson New Zealand Ltd.)
Penguin Books (South Africa) (Pty.) Rosebank Office Park, 181 Jan Smuts Avenue,
Parktown North 2193, South Africa
Penguin China, B7 Jiaming Center, 27 East Third Ring Road North,
Chaoyang District, Beijing 100020, China

Penguin Books Ltd., Registered Offices:
80 Strand, London WC2R 0RL, England

Published by New American Library, a division of Penguin Group (USA) Inc. Previously published in the United Kingdom by Vermilion, an imprint of Ebury Publishing, a Random House company. For information contact The Random House Group, 20 Vauxhall Bridge Road, London, Greater London SW1V 2SA, England.

First New American Library Printing, March 2013
10

REGISTERED TRADEMARK—MARCA REGISTRADA

LIBRARY OF CONGRESS CATALOGING-IN-PUBLICATION DATA:
Ford, Gina.
The new contented little baby book: the secret to calm and confident parenting/Gina Ford.
p. cm.
Rev. ed. of: Contented little baby book/Gina Ford. 1999.
Includes index.
ISBN 978-0-451-41565-3
1. Newborn infants—Care. 2. Newborn infants—Health and hygiene.
3. Newborn infants—Weaning. 4. Parenting. 5. Child rearing.
I. Ford, Gina. Contented little baby book. II. Title.
RJ131.F64 2013
649'.1—dc23   2012027286

Set in Adobe Garamond Pro
Designed by Pauline Neuwirth

Printed in the United States of America

PUBLISHER'S NOTE

Every effort has been made to ensure that the information contained in this book is complete and accurate. However, neither the publisher nor the author is engaged in rendering professional advice or services to the individual reader. The ideas, procedures, and suggestions contained in this book are not intended as a substitute for consulting with your physician. All matters regarding your health require medical supervision. Neither the author nor the publisher shall be liable or responsible for any loss or damage allegedly arising from any information or suggestion in this book. The opinions expressed in this book represent the personal views of the author and not of the publisher.

While the author has made every effort to provide accurate telephone numbers, Internet addresses, and other contact information at the time of publication, neither the publisher nor the author assumes any responsibility for errors, or for changes that occur after publication. Further, publisher does not have any control over and does not assume any responsibility for author or third-party Web sites or their content.

To my beloved mother and best friend in remembrance

of her blessed wisdom, the very special love, support

and encouragement which she always gave me and

whose wonderful smile and sparkling eyes could turn a

rainy day into sunshine.

• Contents •

Contents

Contents

Contents

The New
Contented Little
Baby Book

Introduction

. . . .

My first book, *The Contented Little Baby Book* (first published in 1999), was based on my personal experiences of working with more than 300 babies and their families in many different parts of the world. It became a bestseller and has been used, and continues to be used, by hundreds of thousands of families across five continents.

The popularity of my advice, and loyal support of the book's followers, is testimony that babies can and do thrive very successfully on routines. Unlike the old-fashioned and inflexible every-four-hours routines, my routines are based on a baby's natural feeding and sleeping rhythms, ensuring that a baby's needs are met before he gets distressed or overtired. Most important, the routines can be adapted to suit the individual needs of each baby; from extensive experience, I know that all babies are different.

In the time since my first book was published, I have communicated with thousands of parents as a result of my consultancy work and through the Contented Baby Web site, www.

contentedbaby.com. The regular and direct contact has enabled me to obtain useful feedback from parents on the Contented Little Baby (CLB) routines, which in turn has inspired me to fully revise and update my original book. The CLB routines and my core philosophy remain the same, but my advice has been expanded in response to this valuable feedback and adapted to today's circumstances.

I am confident that this revised book will be even better at teaching you how to recognize the difference between hunger and tiredness, how to establish good feeding and sleeping patterns, and how to meet all of your precious baby's needs. With help from this totally revised edition, becoming a parent should be a happy and deeply satisfying experience for both you and your baby. The CLB routines have worked for many thousands of parents and their contented babies, and they can work for you too.

🎲 1 🎲

Preparation for the Birth

· · · · · ·

When one talks of preparing for the birth, the first things that spring to mind are prenatal care and decorating the nursery. Both are important in their own ways. Prenatal care is of the utmost importance for a healthy pregnancy and helps to prepare you for the birth; and decorating the nursery for the new arrival is fun. While many of the prenatal classes available do give some advice on what is ahead after the birth, they often focus on the birth itself and overlook very practical tips, which, if offered early enough, can save parents hours of time and stress after their baby is born.

If you follow my routines from day one, you should be fortunate enough to have a contented and happy baby, with some time for yourself. However, as you will see from my routines and charts, spare time is extremely limited (and, believe me, mothers who are not following a routine have even less spare time). In this short amount of time, unless you have help, you will have to fit in preparing meals, shopping, laundry, etc.

By doing the following things before the baby is born, you will gain many hours of free time after the birth:

* Order all your nursery equipment well in advance. Cribs can sometimes take up to 12 weeks to be delivered, and there are many advantages in having the crib from the beginning.
* Have all the bed linen, burp cloths and towels washed and ready for use. Purchase the crib, baby carrier and stroller. Prepare everything in the nursery, so it is easy to find when you get home from the hospital.
* Have the following baby essentials in stock: cotton balls, baby oil, diapers, diaper creams, baby wipes, soft sponges, baby hair brush, bath oil and baby shampoo.
* Check that all the electrical equipment is working properly. Learn how the sterilizer works and how to put together the feeding bottles.
* Arrange a section of worktop in the kitchen where preparation and sterilization can be done. Ideally, it should be directly below a cupboard where all of the baby's feeding equipment can be stored.
* Stock up on laundry detergent, cleaning materials and enough paper towels and toilet paper to last at least six weeks.
* Prepare and freeze a large selection of healthy home-made meals for you and your husband/partner. If you are breast-feeding, you should avoid the store-bought meals that are full of additives and preservatives.
* Stock up on extra dry goods such as tea, coffee, crackers, etc.; it is inevitable that you will have extra visitors the first month, and supplies will soon go down.
* Purchase birthday gifts and cards for any forthcoming

birthdays. Also, have a good selection of thank-you cards ready to send for all the gifts you will receive.

✳ Get up to date with any odd jobs that need to be done in the house or garden. The last thing you need once the baby has arrived is the hassle of workers coming and going.

✳ If breast-feeding, purchase your electric breast pump well in advance.

. . . .

The Nursery

Like most parents with a newborn, you will probably have your baby sleeping in your room with you during the night. The current advice from the Academy of American Pediatrics is that your baby should sleep in the same room as you until he is six months old. However, I still believe it is important to have the nursery ready on your return from the hospital. All too often mothers will call me in a complete panic, asking for advice on how to get older babies used to their own room. Many tears and much anxiety could have been avoided if the mothers had gotten their babies used to their own room from day one. Instead, for the first few months, the baby is fed, changed, played with and put to sleep wherever the parents spend their time. It is not surprising that these babies feel abandoned when they are eventually put to sleep by themselves in an unfamiliar, dark room.

From the very beginning, you should use the nursery as much as possible for diaper changing, feeding and some quiet play. By getting your baby used to his room from the beginning, he will very quickly enjoy being there and see it as a peaceful haven.

. . . .

When babies are very small, especially if they have become overtired and overstimulated, it is useful to have a quiet, comfortable room where they can wind down. Using your baby's nursery for this purpose in the early days will help him to make the transition from sleeping in the same room with you to sleeping in his own room, once he reaches six months.

Decoration

It is not essential to spend a fortune on decorating and furnishing the baby's room. A room with walls, windows and bed linen covered in teddy bears soon becomes very boring. Plain walls can easily be brightened with a colorful border and perhaps a matching valance and curtains; this makes it easy to adapt the room as the baby grows but avoids the need to redecorate totally. (Another very cost-effective and fun way to liven up the room is to use sheets of children's wrapping paper as posters, which are bright and colorful—and can be changed frequently.)

The Crib

Most baby books advise that in the early days a crib is not necessary as babies are happier in a baby carrier or bassinet. While it may seem a more practical solution when moving your baby from room to room with you (see Chapter Five, Establishing the Contented Little Baby Routines, for current advice), I am not convinced babies are happier or they sleep better in these. However, since the American Academy of Pediatrics (www.healthychildren.org) recommends that the safest place for your baby to sleep is in your room, the best option appears to be having a bassinet with a firm mattress made up for him that he will use for the duration of this period. As I have said, I much preferred to get my babies used to their big crib from day one so I would recommend allowing your baby to spend some time in his crib, having some quiet play and winding down there after feeding. By doing this, I never encountered a problem when they outgrew their baby carrier and started to sleep the whole night in their big crib in the nursery.

When choosing a crib, it is important to remember that it will be your baby's bed for at least two or three years and should, therefore, be sturdy enough to withstand a bouncing toddler. Even very young babies will eventually move around in their crib.

I suggest choosing a design with flat slats instead of round ones, as pressing the head against a round slat can be quite painful for a young baby. Crib bumpers are not advised for babies less than one year old, as they can end up sleeping with their heads pressed up against the bumpers. Because body heat escapes through the top of the head, blocking it off increases the risk of overheating. This is thought to be a contributing factor in crib death.

Other points to bear in mind when choosing cribs:

* Look for two or three different base height levels.
* Drop-sides should be easy to put up and down without making a noise. Test them several times.
* The crib should be large enough to accommodate a two-year-old child comfortably.
* There should not be too much of a gap around the edges of the mattress and the crib.
* Buy the best mattresses that you can afford. I have found that foam mattresses tend to sink in the middle within a few months. The type I have found to give the

best support for growing babies is an "inner spring" type.

* All cribs and mattresses should comply with the recommendations set by the Consumer Product Safety Commission (www.cpsc.gov/info/cribs).

Bedding for the Crib

Everything should be 100 percent white cotton so that it can be washed in hot water along with the baby's night clothes. Due to the risk of overheating or smothering, quilts and duvets are not recommended for babies less than one year old. If you want a matching top cover for your baby's crib, make sure it is 100 percent cotton and not quilted with a nylon filling. For parents who are handy with a sewing machine, a considerable amount of money can be saved by making flat and draw sheets (flat sheets that go crosswise across the top end of the bottom sheet) out of a double- or queen-size sheet.

You will need at least the following bedding:

* Three stretch-cotton fitted bottom sheets. Choose the soft jersey-type cotton rather than the toweling type, which can very quickly become rough and worn-looking.
* Three flat, smooth cotton top sheets. Avoid flannel, which gives off too much fluff for young babies; this can obstruct the nose and cause breathing problems.
* Three cotton, small-weave cellular blankets, plus one wool blanket for very cold nights.
* Six flat, smooth cotton bassinet sheets. These are small sheets that are used for bassinets and baby carriers but are also ideal as draw sheets, which you should put across the head end of the bottom sheet. This elimi-

nates the need to remake the whole crib in the middle of the night or during naps, should your baby dribble or his diaper leak.

MAKING UP THE CRIB

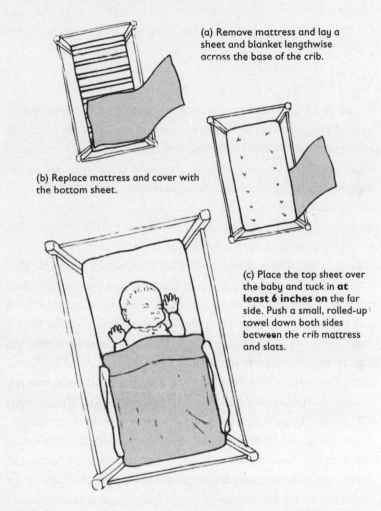

(a) Remove mattress and lay a sheet and blanket lengthwise across the base of the crib.

(b) Replace mattress and cover with the bottom sheet.

(c) Place the top sheet over the baby and tuck in **at least 6 inches on** the far side. Push a small, rolled-up towel down both sides between the crib mattress and slats.

Changing Station

The most practical changing station is a long unit, containing drawers and a cupboard. The surface should be large enough to hold both the changing mat and the washbowl. The drawers can be used to store pajamas, underwear and burp cloths, and the cupboard can hold larger items, such as diaper packs.

Wardrobe

A built-in closet is a very good investment for your nursery as it enables you to keep the baby's clothes tidy and crease-free, and it will provide valuable storage space for the many pieces of equipment that you will accumulate. If a built-in is out of the question, purchase a dresser or armoire.

Chair

It is essential, no matter how small your baby's room is, that you fit in a chair. A sturdy comfortable chair is an absolute priority. A small two-seater pull-out sleep sofa is a good choice as it can be used for both feeding and for sleeping in the baby's room. If space is limited, then choose a chair with a straight back. It should be wide enough to allow room for you and your baby as he grows, and, ideally, the arms should be wide enough to support you while breast-feeding. I would resist the temptation to buy a rocking chair, which is often sold as a nursing chair. These can be dangerous as the baby becomes more mobile and may attempt to pull himself up by holding onto the chair. In the early days, it can also be tempting to settle your baby by rocking him to sleep, but this is one of the main causes of a baby developing poor sleeping habits.

Curtains

Curtains should be full-length and fully lined with blackout lining (see Useful Addresses in the back of the book). Fix them to a track that fits flush along the top of the window. Ideally, they should have a deep matching valance, which is also lined with blackout lining. There should be no gaps between the sides of the curtains and the window frame; even the smallest chink of light can be enough to wake your baby earlier than 7 a.m. For the same reason, curtain rods should be avoided as light streams through the gap at the top. As your baby gets older, he may not settle back to sleep if woken at 5 a.m. by early-morning sun in the summer or by streetlights.

When the lights are off and the curtains are closed, it should be so dark that you are unable to see your partner standing at the other side of the room. Research has shown that the chemicals in the brain alter in the dark, conditioning the body for sleep.

Carpeting

Wall-to-wall carpet is preferable to scatter or area rugs, which you might trip on when you are attending to your baby in dim light. Consider choosing a carpet that is treated with a stainguard, and avoid very dark or bright colors, as they tend to show dirt more easily.

Lighting

If the main light in the nursery is not already fitted with a dimmer switch, it would be worthwhile changing it. In the early days, dimming the lights when settling the baby is a good association signal. If you are on a limited budget, purchase one of the small plug-in night-lights that fit into any normal electrical socket.

· · · · · · · · · · · ·

Baby Equipment

Baby Carrier or Small Crib

As I mentioned earlier, a baby carrier is not essential. Even the cheapest of baby carriers and a stand can cost more than fifty dollars, which is quite a lot of money for something that your baby will outgrow within six weeks. However, if you live in a very large house or plan to travel in the first few weeks, a baby carrier's portability may make it a worthwhile purchase. If your budget is limited, try to borrow one from a friend and buy a new mattress.

A bassinet is a small version of a full-sized crib. Certainly, it is bigger than a baby carrier, but not really any more practical. Because we now put our babies to sleep on their back, these bassinets create a problem for small babies. They can wake themselves up several times a night because the mattresses are not wide enough for them to sleep with their arms stretched out fully, and they can get their hands caught between the slats.

If you do decide to use either of these items for a short period, you will need the following bedding:

* Three fitted, stretch cotton bottom sheets. Choose the soft, smooth jersey-type cotton.
* Six smooth cotton flat sheets, to be used as top sheets and later as draw sheets on the big crib.
* Four cotton, cellular close-weave bassinet blankets.

· · · · ·

✳ A dozen burp cloths to be placed across the top or bottom of the bassinet or crib to catch dribbles and diaper leaks.

Stroller

There are several types of transport you can choose: a single-function stroller, a jogging stroller or a combination stroller and bassinet/car seat, to name a few. When choosing one of these, it is important to take into consideration that your baby will sleep in it for parts of the day until he is six months old. It is also important to take into consideration where you live and your lifestyle. For example, if you have to drive to the nearest store, it is important to choose a stroller that is easy to open and close and is not too heavy to lift in and out of the car. There are now some very lightweight strollers on the market that recline flat for a newborn baby, and come with a hood and apron designed to give the baby some protection from the sun and also the rain and cold.

The "three-in-one," a travel system that can be used with a bassinet in the early days and later with a car seat, can be a very good choice if you live in a quieter area and can walk to where you need to go.

If you are likely to be using your stroller in an urban area or in stores with narrow aisles, swivel wheels are a must. They make turning the stroller around corners effortless compared to what it would be with set wheels.

Whichever type you choose, you should practice putting it up and down several times and try lifting it onto a surface in the store to get an idea of how easy it is going to be to lift into the car.

The following guidelines should also be followed when purchasing any kind of stroller:

* It should be fitted with good, strong safety straps that go over the baby's shoulders as well as around the waist, and have an easy-to-operate brake.
* Make sure it has a hood and apron to protect the baby from the elements.
* Buy all the extras at the same time: sun canopy, rain cover, foot cover, head-support cushion and shopping tray or bag. Models often change in design and sometimes dimension, and if you wait until next season, the items you require might not fit or match.
* Try pushing the stroller around the store to check if the handle height is at a comfortable level; also observe how easily it moves in and out of doorways and round corners.

Car Seat

You will need to have a backward-facing car seat to bring your baby home from the hospital. An infant car seat should always be used, even on short journeys. Never be tempted to travel holding your baby in your arms as it's against the law! In the event of a collision or emergency stop, it would be impossible to keep hold of your baby. Car seats should not be fitted to the front passenger seat if the car has airbags, unless these have been adequately disabled. Follow the current safety regulations and check the National Highway Traffic Safety Administration Web site (www.nhtsa.gov) for up-to-date laws and regulations. In general, choose the best car seat you can afford and preferably one that comes with clear instructions for installation.

Other things to look for include the following:

* A seat with large side wings, which offer more protection in a side-impact collision.

✳ A five-point harness, which will make it much easier to adjust the seat to your baby's clothing.
✳ A buckle that is easy for an adult, but not a child, to open and close.
✳ The availability of extra accessories, such as a head-support pillow or replacement cover.

Baby Bath

A baby bath is another item that is not essential. Like the baby carrier or the bassinet, babies outgrow the small bath very quickly. A newborn baby can be bathed in a sink to begin with or even in a bathtub using one of the several types of bath seats that are available for tiny babies. These allow the baby to lie supported and on a slight slope, leaving the caregiver with both hands free to wash the baby.

If you would feel more confident with a special baby bath, the one I would recommend is designed to fit across a big bath. It makes filling and emptying much easier, unlike the bath that is incorporated into a changing station. I have found these totally impractical because, as you lift the baby out of the bath, you have to maneuver the lid, which doubles as the changing table, down over the top of the bath before you can put the baby on it to dry and dress him. They are also very difficult to empty; I found I always had to tip the whole thing on its side to drain the water out completely. This usually ends up with all the items stored below toppling onto the floor. These bath/changing stations are very expensive, and I would discourage anyone from buying them.

Changing Mat

It is worthwhile to buy two changing mats. Choose easy-clean plastic with well-padded sides. In the early days, it is best to lay a hand towel on the top, as very young babies hate to be laid down on anything cold.

Baby Monitor

This is an important piece of equipment, so don't skimp when buying it. There are generally two types to choose from, plug-in and mobile, but I would advise you to look at the mobile version that allows you to move freely around the house, including areas such as the bathroom, which might not have an electrical socket for the plug-in version. There is a growing body of scientific evidence to suggest that digital (or DECT) monitors expose babies to more pulsing microwave radiation than cell phone base station masts. For this reason, I recommend that you choose an analogue baby monitor.

When choosing a baby monitor, look for the following features:

* A visual display as well as sound, which allows you to monitor your baby even with the volume turned down.
* Monitors work using radio frequencies, so choose a model with two channels, which allows you to switch channels if there is interference.
* A rechargeable model is more expensive initially, but the saving on batteries will make it cheaper in the long run.
* A low-battery indicator and an out-of-range indicator.

Baby Sling

Some parents swear by this method of moving around with their babies. I never use one as I find it too big a strain on my back to carry a baby around like this for any length of time. Very small babies are also inclined to go straight to sleep the minute you hold them close to your chest, which defeats the whole purpose of my routines—i.e. keeping the baby awake at certain times of the day, and teaching the baby the right associations for going to sleep on his own. I do think that as babies get bigger, slings are a very useful way for parents to carry them around, especially when the baby is old enough to face outward.

If you feel a sling would be useful, here are some guidelines to observe when choosing one:

* The sling must have safety tabs to ensure it cannot come undone.
* It must provide your baby with enough head and neck support; some come with a detachable cushion that gives extra support for very young babies.
* It should offer the choice of baby facing inward or outward and have a seat with an adjustable height position.
* It should be made of strong, washable fabric with comfortable, padded shoulder straps.
* I would certainly recommend trying it on in the store and putting a baby into it—one size does not fit all!

Baby Chair

While many parents use a car seat in the house for their baby to sit in during the day, if your budget will stretch, having a second seat for your baby can be a great bonus as it saves having to move the seat from room to room.

Baby seats come in different styles. Some chairs are rigid, with adjustable seat positions and a base that can either remain stable or be set to rocking mode. Another type is known as a "bouncy chair." This type is made of a lightweight frame covered in fabric and is designed to bounce as the baby moves. I have found them to be very popular with babies more than two months old, but they can make tiny babies feel insecure. Whatever type of chair you choose, make sure your baby is securely strapped in and never left unattended. Also, always place the baby on the floor when she is in a seat; never be tempted to leave her on a table or worktop, as the movement of the baby can easily shift the chair to the edge.

Here are some further guidelines:

* The frame and base should be firm and sturdy and fitted with a strong safety strap.
* Choose one with an easily removable and washable cover.
* Buy a head support cushion for tiny babies.

Playpen

Playpens are frowned upon by some "baby experts," who feel they hinder a baby's natural instinct to explore. My own feeling is that, while babies should never be left for long periods in a playpen, they can be very useful for making sure that your child is safe when you need to do something else. If you do decide to use a playpen, I would recommend getting your baby used to it from a young age. A pack-and-play can be used as a playpen, but if you have the space, I recommend the square wooden type, which is larger and enables your baby to pull himself up and move around. Whichever sort you choose, make sure it is situated out of reach of hazards such as radiators, curtains and trailing electrical wires. Never hang toys on pieces of string or cord in the playpen, as these could prove fatal if your baby were to get tangled in one.

Important points to look for when choosing a playpen:

* Make sure it has a fixed floor so that your baby cannot move it.
* Check that there are no sharp metal hinges or catches on which your baby could harm himself.
* If choosing a mesh-type playpen or travel crib, make sure that the mesh is strong enough to prevent your baby pushing small toys through and making a hole big enough to trap his hand or fingers.

. . . .

Equipment Needed for Breast-feeding

Nursing Bra

These are bras made with specially designed cups that can either be unhooked or unzipped to make breast-feeding easier. Whatever style of bra you choose, it should fit well. A good nursing bra should be made of cotton for comfort, have wide, adjustable shoulder straps to help support your breasts and should not press tightly against the nipples, as this can be a cause of blocked milk ducts. I suggest buying two nursing bras before the birth. If they prove comfortable after your milk has come in, you can buy more.

. . . . .

Breast Pads

In the early days, you will use a lot of breast pads, as they need to be changed every time after your baby feeds. Many mothers prefer the round ones, contoured to fit the breasts. You may need to experiment with different brands, but sometimes the more expensive ones have better absorbency, so they offer better value in the long run.

Nursing Pillow

These pillows are shaped to fit around a mother's waist, bringing small babies up to the perfect height for breast-feeding. They can also be used for propping babies up and make an excellent back support for older babies who are learning to sit up. If you decide to invest in one, make sure it has a removable, machine-washable cover.

Nipple Cream and Sprays

These are designed to care for the breasts and help relieve any pain caused by breast-feeding. The main cause of pain, however, is poor positioning of the baby on the breast. If you experience pain either during or after feeding, it would be wise to consult your doctor or lactation consultant for advice before purchasing a cream or spray. No other special creams or soaps are recommended when breast-feeding. Simply wash your breasts twice a day with plain water and after each feeding. The nipples should be rubbed with a little breast milk and allowed to air dry.

Electric Breast Pump

I am convinced that one of the reasons the majority of mothers I advise are successful at breast-feeding is because I encourage the use of an electric breast pump. In the very early days when you are producing more milk than your baby may need (especially first thing in the morning), this milk can be expressed using one of these powerful machines. The expressed milk can then be stored in the fridge or freezer and used as a top-up later in the day when you are tired and your milk supply may be low. Not enough milk is, I believe, one of the main reasons why so many babies are restless and will not settle after their bath in the evening. If you want to breast-feed and quickly establish your baby in a routine, an electric breast pump will be a big asset. Do not be tempted by one of the smaller hand versions, which can be so inefficient as to put many women off expressing at all.

Freezer Bags

Expressed milk can be stored in the fridge for up to twenty-four hours or in the freezer for one month. Specially designed, presterilized bags are an ideal way to store expressed breast milk and are available from chemists or baby departments in the larger stores.

Bottles

Most lactation consultants are against newborn babies being given a bottle, even of expressed milk. They claim that it creates nipple confusion, reducing the baby's desire to suck on the breast, leading in turn to poor milk supply and the mother giving up breast-feeding altogether. My own view is that the majority of women give up breast-feeding because they are totally exhausted with "demand feeding," often several times a night. I advise giving babies a bottle a day of either expressed milk or formula milk from the first week and introducing it by the fourth week at the latest. This one bottle can be given either last thing in the evening or during the night by someone other than the mother, thereby allowing the mother to sleep for several hours at a stretch. This, in turn, is likely to make her more able to cope with breast-feeding. I have never had a problem with a baby rejecting the mother's breast or becoming confused between breast nipple and bottle nipple, but this could happen if, in the early days, a baby was offered more than one bottle a day. Other good reasons for getting your baby used to a bottle are the following: first, it gives you some flexibility; second, the problem of later introducing bottles to an exclusively breast-fed baby doesn't arise; and third, it gives the baby's father a wonderful opportunity to become more involved.

There are many types of bottles available, all claiming to be the best. From experience, I always recommend a wide-necked design as it makes cleaning and filling easier. It is also worth looking around for bottles that are free of Bisphenol A (BPA) as some scientists believe that this chemical, common in clear plastic feeding bottles, can leach into the milk.

I suggest that you start by using a newborn nipple, which will encourage your baby to work as hard drinking milk from a bottle as when breast-feeding. However, using a nipple that is too slow for your baby can lead to problems such as wind, so take your baby's lead on this and move on to a faster-flowing one as soon as he seems to struggle—this may be as early as three weeks but usually occurs around the eight-week mark. For advice on sterilizing equipment, please refer to the next section.

. . . .

Equipment Needed for Bottle-feeding

Bottles

For the reasons already mentioned, I strongly advise buying the wide-necked bottles described previously. If your baby is likely to take all his milk from a bottle, it is important that the risk of developing colic or wind is kept to a minimum. When called upon to help a baby with colic, I often see an immediate improvement simply by switching to these wide-necked bottles. The nipple is designed to be flexible, and it allows the baby to suckle as he would at the breast. The wide-necked bottles, in time, can also be adapted to become feeding cups with soft spouts and handles. If your baby is being exclusively bottle-fed, I advise that you start with five 8-oz. bottles and three 4-oz. bottles.

Nipples

Most bottles come with a slow-flow nipple designed to meet the needs of newborns. By eight weeks, I have found that most babies feed better from a medium-flow nipple, and it is worthwhile stocking up on these extra nipples from the beginning.

Bottle Brush

Complete and thorough cleaning of your baby's bottles is of the utmost importance. Choose a brush with an extra-long plastic handle, which will allow more force to be put into cleaning the bottles.

Nipple Brush

Most mothers find that the easiest way to clean a nipple is by using their forefinger. However, if you have extra-long nails, it may be worth investing in a nipple brush, although they too can damage the hole of the nipple, resulting in the need to replace the nipples more frequently. Short nails are probably the answer!

Washing-up Bowl

It is easier to organize and keep track of what is sterilized if all the dirty bottles are washed and sterilized at the same time. You will need somewhere to put the rinsed-out bottles and nipples until they are ready to be sterilized, and a large stainless steel or plastic bowl can be used for this purpose, preferably with a lid.

Sterilizer

Whether you are breast- or bottle-feeding, it is essential that all bottles and expressing equipment be sterilized properly. Most U.S. agencies say that washing bottles and nipples in the hot cycle of the dishwasher is satisfactory. For those who question the purity of their water or prefer to be more vigilant, there are three main methods of sterilization: boiling equipment for ten minutes in a large pan; soaking equipment in a sterilizing solution for two hours and rinsing with boiling-hot water; or using an electric steam sterilizer. From experience, I can say that the easiest, fastest and most effective method is the steam sterilizer, and it is well worth making this investment. A word of caution— don't be tempted to purchase a microwave version. This type of unit holds fewer bottles, and it becomes a complete nuisance when you have to remove it to use the microwave for other purposes.

Kettle

Obviously, a kettle is essential for mixing formula, so it should be efficient and of sufficient size. If you decide to formula-feed right from the beginning, you will spend a lot of time in the first year making formulas. The water for the formula needs to be fresh, boiled just once and cooled before the powder is added. If you don't already have an extra kettle, you might consider investing in one. If you're expecting twins, it is essential.

Bottle Insulator

This is a special type of thermos designed to keep bottles of boiled water warm. It can be very useful when traveling, or for mixing nighttime feedings quickly.

Clothes for the Newborn

The range of infant wear available in stores is both delightful and bewildering. While it can be fun choosing garments for your baby, I urge you to approach this particular area with caution. Newborn babies grow at an alarming rate and will outgrow most of their first-size clothes by the first month, unless they were very small at birth. Although it is important to have enough clothes to allow for frequent changing, if you have too many, most will never be worn. You will need to renew your baby's wardrobe at least three times in the first year, and even if you stick to the cheaper ranges, it will still be a costly business. I advise that you buy only the basics before your baby arrives. You may receive clothing as gifts, and you will have plenty of opportunity for clothes shopping during the first year.

When choosing clothes for the first month, don't be tempted by brightly colored underwear or sleepwear. Newborn babies have a tendency to leak from both ends, and it is impossible to remove stains by washing at anything less than the hottest wash cycle. Brightly colored garments will soon fade if frequently washed at this temperature, so stick to white, and leave the brighter colors for the outer garments.

In general, keep clothing simple during the first month. Dressing your baby in little white socks and onesies in the early days makes washing so much easier. A clothes dryer means that you do not have to worry about ironing if you remove everything from the dryer the minute it is dry. Listed below are the basic items you will need for the first couple of months. Until your baby arrives, I advise against removing packaging or tags, so the items can be exchanged if your baby is either larger or smaller than expected.

Onesies	6–8	Socks	2–3 pairs
Nightdresses or sleep suits	4–6	Hats	2
Day outfits	4–6	Mittens	2 pairs
Sweaters	2–3	Receiving blankets	3
Snowsuit for a winter baby	1	Jacket	1

Onesies

A newborn baby would normally wear a one piece in both winter and summer, except in very hot weather. The best fabric next to a baby's skin is 100 percent cotton, and if you want your beautiful layette to retain its appearance after numerous hot washes, stick to plain white, or white with a pale color pattern. The best style of onesie to buy is a "body suit," that fastens under your baby's legs, has short sleeves and an envelope-style neckline for easy dressing.

Nightwear

The most common type of sleepwear is an all-in-one suit, or onesie. They are snug and save time on laundry, but they can be awkward if you have to struggle to get your otherwise settled baby out of one to change his diaper. For this reason, some mothers prefer sleepers, dress-like outfits with easy access to baby's lower half. As with onesies, 100 percent cotton is best, and the simpler the design, the better. Avoid anything with ties at the neck; and if there are ties at the bottom, remove them as they could get caught around your baby's feet.

Day Outfits

During the first couple of months, the easiest thing to dress your baby in will be onesies, which usually come in packs of two or three. Again, choose pure cotton and a style that opens either across the back or inside the legs, to ensure you don't need to undress your baby fully at every diaper change. Dungaree style clothes, without feet and with matching T-shirts, are also useful. They will last a bit longer as your baby grows, and the tops can be interchanged if your baby dribbles a lot. Choose styles in soft cotton knits for very young babies, rather than stiff cotton or denim.

Sweaters

If your baby is born in the summer, you can probably get away with just two sweaters, ideally in cotton. With a winter baby, it is best to have at least three sweaters, preferably wool. As long as your baby has cotton garments next to his skin, there should be no cause for irritation, and the simpler the design, the better.

Socks

Simple socks in cotton or wool are the most practical for new babies. Fancy styles with ribbons should be avoided, as should any type of shoe. However cute they may be, they can harm your baby's soft bones.

Hats

In the summer, it is important that you buy a cotton hat with a brim to protect your baby's head and face from the sun. Ideally, the brim should go right round the back of the neck. In spring and autumn, knitted cotton hats are adequate on cooler days. During the winter, or on very cold days, I suggest a warm wool or fleece hat. Many of these are lined with cotton, but if not, a thin cotton hat can be worn underneath to protect sensitive skin.

Mittens

Small babies do not like to have their hands covered up, as they use them extensively to touch, feel and explore everything in close contact. If, however, your baby has sharp nails or tends to scratch, you could try fine cotton mitts to protect his skin. In very cold weather use woolen or fleece mitts, but again, put cotton ones underneath if your baby has sensitive skin.

Receiving Blanket

I firmly believe that during the first few weeks all babies sleep better when swaddled. Whether you choose a blanket or receiving blanket to swaddle, it should always be made of lightweight pure cotton that has a slight stretch to it. To avoid overheating, always swaddle your baby in a single layer, and reduce the number of blankets on the crib. It is, however, important that by six weeks you start to get your baby used to being half-swaddled, under the arms. Crib death rates peak between two and four months and overheating is thought to be a major factor. Always check that you are not putting too many layers on and that there is sufficient ventilation as recommended by the Academy of American Pediatrics.

Snowsuit

When choosing snowsuits for your baby, always buy at least two sizes too big, as this allows plenty of room for growth. Avoid fancy designs with fur around the hood or dangling toggles, opting instead for one in an easy-care, washable fabric. For tiny babies, buttons may be preferable to a zipper, which can dig into the chin.

Jacket

A lightweight jacket can be useful for babies born at any time of the year. In summer, a jacket can be worn on chilly days, and in winter, on milder ones. As with the snowsuits, choose one in a simple design in a washable fabric.

HOW TO SWADDLE YOUR BABY

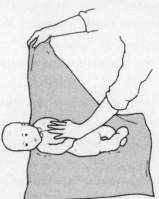

(a) Place baby on square receiving blanket and lift one side, level with back of the head.

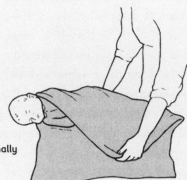

(b) Bring it down diagonally over the shoulder.

(c) Lift the other side up, making it taut.

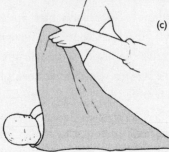

(d) Lift the baby a little and secure the end beneath his body.

. . . .

Your Baby's Laundry

After you have spent a considerable amount of time and money on your baby's wardrobe, it is well worth your effort to be very fussy about caring for it. Because young babies grow out of their clothes so quickly, it should be possible, with good laundering, to pass them on to any brother or sister that follows.

The following guidelines will help keep your baby's laundry in great shape:

* Laundry should be sorted into different-colored piles.
* Bedding, burp cloths and bibs need to be washed on a very hot wash cycle to get rid of bacteria caused by milk stains and to eliminate the house dust mite, which can trigger allergies in very young babies.
* Load the washing machine no more than two-thirds full so that the clothes are rinsed thoroughly.
* Stains should always be treated before washing.

Whites: Hot

Anything that is stained—burp cloths, sheets, onesies, bibs, socks, sleepers—should be soaked overnight in a prewash solution and then washed in a washing machine on hot. Everything should be 100 percent cotton, and bibs or towels with a colored trim should have been tested for running colors by washing separately for the first few washes. Towels and facecloths should be washed and dried together and separate from other clothes, in order to avoid pilling.

Light Colors: Warm

Most day clothes need only a very quick wash in the wool or delicate cycle. Anything stained should be soaked first overnight in prewash and rinsed before washing.

Dark Colors: Cold

Any dark outfits must be washed separately from the light colors even if they do not run; to mix the two will only result in the lighter colors taking on a gray tinge. Anything stained should be soaked first overnight in prewash.

Woolens or Delicates: Handwash

Even if the label says Machine Wash, it is better to handwash using a very small amount of gentle soap mixed with lukewarm water. Always squeeze the garment gently in the water when washing and rinsing; never wring, twist or allow a delicate garment to hang down. Rinse thoroughly in cold running water, gently squeeze out excess water, then roll in a clean, dry, white towel for a few hours. Finally, gently pull into shape and either dry flat or hang across a drying screen. Never hang up woolens from the bottom.

Use of the Clothes Dryer

Towels, bibs, crib sheets and blankets can be tumble-dried. Avoid drying towels and clothes together as it causes pilling. Remove all clothes from the dryer and fold them as soon as possible to avoid wrinkling, and ensure that all clothes are properly aired.

Corduroy and Dark Clothes

To avoid fading, dry these on the cool cycle for no more than 15 minutes. Then pull the clothes into shape and place them on hangers to dry. In this way, they may not need to be ironed.

2

Why Follow a Routine?

· · · · · · ·

Many years have passed since I first typed the four words, "Why follow a routine?" Little did I know then the controversy those four simple words would create. But here I am still, explaining again why I think routine is important. I must stress that my views have not changed one little bit from when I wrote my first book. I personally believe that the majority of babies thrive and are happier in a routine. But I certainly realize and respect that following a routine is not the best choice for all parents.

There is already so much advice out there for "baby-led parenting"; therefore, the advice I give in my books is for those parents who believe that they and their baby will be happier with more structure. I assume that one of the reasons you are reading this book is that you already have a certain level of structure in your life and that you believe you will cope with your baby better by following some sort of routine. If this is the case then I can assure you that following Contented Little Baby routines will most certainly benefit both you and your baby. They are followed successfully by hundreds of thousands of parents around the world. Follow your own instinct as a parent as to what works best for you and your baby; use the routines and advice in this book as tools to help you be the parents that you want to be.

. . . .

Why the CLB Routines Are Different

During the years that I worked as a maternity nurse, I read hundreds of books on child care. I have also had the unique privilege of working personally with more than 300 families around the world. It is because of these parents and their beautiful babies that I feel I am able to share with you so much of what I have learned, which I hope will help you overcome many of the everyday challenges of parenting.

I would typically arrive at a home a few days after the birth and live with the family 24/7 for periods of 3–5 days, or sometimes several weeks to six months. While the media make much of the fact that many of my clients were rich and famous, I can assure you that most of the families I helped were not. They often had to get outside help because of health issues, family bereavement or other personal circumstances. Whether they lived in a mansion with 20 bedrooms or a walk-up apartment with only one bedroom, were a rock or movie star, struggling actor, high-profile banker or teacher, these parents all had two things in common—they wanted to ensure that their baby was happy and contented and that they could manage to meet all of their baby's needs as well as cope with the demanding lives they led.

When I started, the leading child-care books all endorsed baby-led parenting and claimed that it was impossible to put a

. . . . .

small baby into a routine. The implication was that if parents even attempted to do so, they could seriously damage the child's health.

In my first book I said that, having successfully spent many years teaching parents how to put their newborns into a routine that results in a happy, thriving, contented baby, I can only assume that the authors of these books have not personally worked with enough babies to know this is possible. The fact that *The Contented Little Baby Book* became a runaway bestseller through personal recommendation is proof enough that the statement I made in my first edition in 1999 has been proved true.

Parents who have properly read the book, the routines and the advice I give can testify that the CLB routines really do work. Unlike old-fashioned every-four-hours feeding, they do not involve leaving a baby to yell until a feeding is due or letting him cry himself to sleep for lengthy periods. While establishing a routine is often very hard work and requires sacrifices on the part of the parents, hundreds of thousands of parents around the world will testify that it is worth it because they quickly learn how to meet the needs of their babies so that any distress is kept to a minimum.

Benefits for Your Baby

The reason that the CLB routines are different from traditional every-four-hours routines is that they are created to meet the natural sleep and feeding needs of all normal, healthy babies. They also allow for some babies needing more sleep than others and some going longer between feedings than others. The aim of the routines is not to push your baby through the night without a feeding but to ensure that structuring his eating and sleeping during the day will keep his nighttime waking at a minimum. He will wake and eat quickly before settling back to sleep. The routines also ensure that once your baby is capable of going longer between feedings, this will happen in the middle of the night, not during the day. The basis of these routines evolved over many years of observing babies in my care. Some babies would develop an eating pattern very quickly with little prompting, while others would be difficult to feed and settle for many weeks.

The following are the main observations that I made from babies who settled into a pattern quickly:

* The parents had a positive approach, wanted a routine and tried to keep the first couple of weeks as calm as possible.
* Handling of the baby by visitors was kept to a minimum so that the baby felt relaxed and secure in his new surroundings (which is especially important when the baby is first brought home from the hospital).
* The baby always had regular sleep times in a quiet room.
* The baby was kept awake for a short spell after the daytime feedings.
* When he was awake and had been well fed and winded, he was then stimulated and played with for short periods.
* A bedtime routine was established from day one. He would be bathed at the same time every evening, then fed and settled in a quiet room. If the baby did not settle, the parents would ensure that they kept things as quiet as possible and continued to comfort him in a dimly lit room until he did eventually settle.

. . . .

Benefits for You

Listening to their baby crying is stressful for parents, particularly if the crying goes on for any length of time despite all their attempts to calm him. By following the CLB routines, you will soon learn the signs of hunger, tiredness, boredom and many other reasons why young babies get upset. The fact that you are able to understand his needs and meet them quickly and confidently will leave both you and your baby calm and reassured and avoid unnecessary crying. The common situation of fretful baby and anxious parents is avoided.

The other big plus for parents following my routines is that they have free time in the evening to relax and enjoy each other's company. This is not usually possible for parents who follow baby-led parenting, as any attachment parenting Web site will show the early evening is a time when these babies are often particularly fretful and require endless rocking and patting to try to keep them calm.

. . . .

Other Approaches

The routines and advice in this book evolved over many years. During my time as a maternity nurse, I tried and tested various ways of establishing breast-feeding and healthy sleep habits. Before I further expand on why I believe my methods are so successful, I will briefly discuss the other methods I have had experience with over the years, which I hope will give you an insight into why I believe that the CLB routines can be of great benefit to today's readers.

. . . . .

Strict Every-Four-Hours-Feeding Routine

This routine evolved when hospital birth took over from home delivery many decades ago, and women would stay in the maternity unit for up to 10–14 days. Their babies were brought to them from the nursery every four hours and given a strict 10–15 minutes on each breast before being returned to the nursery. Although such routines are more associated with our grandmothers' generation, there are still parents nowadays who believe that babies can be slotted into them. During my early years of working as a maternity nurse, I did work with some families that adopted these routines and, for some babies they did succeed, particularly if they were formula-fed.

However, I did find that trying to establish breast-feeding with a strict every-four-hours schedule, in which feedings were limited to a strict 10–15 minutes on each breast, did not work for most babies. The mother, believing that the reason her baby was not managing to stick to the schedule was because she was not producing enough milk, would be pressured early on to introduce top-up feedings of formula in order to get the baby to nurse at the right times according to the routines. I would be a multimillionaire if I had a dollar for every grandmother who said to me, "My milk dried up the minute I left the hospital." The reality was that, due to rigid routines and restricted timing of feedings, the mother's milk had started to dry up long before she left the hospital. The trend for bottle-feeding became well established in the 1950s and 1960s, with many mothers not even attempting to breast-feed. This trend continued well into the 1970s. Then, as research started to unearth more and more information regarding the health benefits of breast-feeding, the trend started to swing back again. Mothers were told not to restrict feedings and to allow their babies to nurse for as long as was needed to satisfy their hunger.

The CLB routines are not about strict four-hour-feeding schedules. It might be many weeks before an every-four-hours pattern can emerge, and I urge you not to be pressured into it, however keen you are to establish a routine. The main reasons every-four-hours feeding can fail:

* Six feedings a day in the early days are usually not enough to stimulate a good milk supply.
* Babies need to nurse little and often in the early days; restricting him to six feedings a day may lead to his being short of his daily intake.
* Babies between one week and six weeks old usually need at least 30 minutes to reach the hind milk.
* Hind milk is at least three times higher in fat content than fore milk and is essential for satisfying your baby's hunger.

Demand Feeding

Although I did look after some babies that were put on a strict every-four-hours-feeding routine from birth, much of my experience in the early days of my career was with babies who were being fed on demand.

The advice given then is the same nowadays. Mothers are encouraged to let their babies take the lead, allowing them to nurse as often and for as long as they want. This method, like the every-four-hours method of feeding, did succeed for some babies, but it did not work for a huge number that I was asked to help. Very early in my experience, it became obvious that, quite simply, many newborn babies do not demand to be fed. This is particularly true of low-birth-weight babies and twins.

That is my main objection to demand feeding. If you had

had the experience of sitting by the bedside of a baby only days old, fighting for his life because he has become seriously dehydrated through not being fed enough, you would probably feel the same way. Dehydration is a very serious problem among newborn babies and one that many new parents are now aware.

The production of breast milk works on a supply-and-demand basis, so babies who are allowed to sleep for long periods between feedings are not put to the breast often enough in a 24-hour period to signal the breasts to make enough milk. Mothers are lulled into a false sense of security that they have a baby who is easy and sleeps well.

In fact, what they have is a very sleepy baby who normally, 2–3 weeks down the line, will start waking more often and demanding more milk than the mother is producing. A pattern quickly emerges of the baby having to feed every couple of hours, day and night, in order to meet his daily nutritional needs.

The current advice is that this pattern is normal and that the baby will sort itself out, but mothers are not told that with some babies it may take months! Sometimes a pattern does emerge in which the baby will go longer between feedings. But often the baby is eating so much in the night that when he does wake for feedings during the day, they tend to be short and small. This leads to a vicious circle of the baby needing to feed more in the night to satisfy his daily needs. The mother then becomes exhausted. This exhaustion can often lead to some or all of the following problems:

✳ Exhaustion and stress reduce the mother's milk supply, increasing the baby's need to nurse little and often.

✳ Babies who continue to need to nurse 10–12 times a

day after the first week often become so exhausted from lack of quality sleep that they become even more tired and feed for shorter and shorter periods.

✳ Exhaustion can lead to the mother getting sick.

✳ Being too tired to concentrate properly can lead to positioning the baby incorrectly on the breast. Poor positioning is the main reason for painful and often cracked and bleeding nipples, which again reduces how well the baby feeds at the breast.

✳ A sleepy baby left too long between feedings in the early days reduces the mother's chances of building up a good milk supply.

Another reason I am so opposed to the term *demand feeding* is that it is often taken too literally. If the baby is fed every time he cries, mothers tend not to look for other reasons as to why the baby may be crying—overstimulation or overtiredness, for example.

Of course, all babies must be fed if they are genuinely hungry; no baby should have to cry to be fed or should be kept on a strict timetable if he is genuinely hungry. But in my experience, and if research on sleeping problems is anything to go by, a huge number of demand-fed babies do not automatically fall into a healthy sleeping pattern months down the line. Many continue to wake and feed little and often long after they are capable of going a longer spell in the night. Another problem is that babies who continue to feed little and often invariably end up being fed to sleep. This creates a whole other set of sleeping problems, in which they have learned the wrong sleep associations and cannot get to sleep without being nursed.

Whether you are the parent of a newborn baby or of an older baby, I urge you not even to attempt to start the routines until you have read and understood Chapters Three, Milk Feeding in the First Year, and Four, Understanding Your Baby's Sleep, on feeding and sleeping in the first year. Because CLB routines are not like the old-fashioned every-four-hours routines, it is not just a case of trying to fit your baby's feeding and sleeping into the times I suggest. The CLB routines change ten times during the first year. The times given for feeding and sleeping in each set of the routines are approximate guidelines for your baby's age, not rigid rules. You need to understand the principles behind the routines so that you can make necessary adjustments to ensure that your baby's individual needs are being met.

. . . .

Your Questions Answered

Q I am six months pregnant, and like many new mothers-to-be, I am concerned about how I am going to cope with the sleepless nights. My prenatal class stresses the importance of demand feeding, that new babies should be fed when they need it and that I should not attempt a routine in the early days. I am concerned that if I try to follow your routines, I may be denying my baby food when he is hungry.

A The CLB routines are not about denying babies food when they are hungry. Quite the opposite. My main concern about demand feeding with very young babies is that a great many babies do not demand to be fed in the very early days. This can lead to many serious problems, the main one being that a baby who is not feeding from the breast will not stimulate the breast to produce enough milk. We, therefore, arrive at the situation,

. . . . .

three or four weeks down the line, in which a mother is trying to feed her baby and not producing enough milk. A vicious circle then evolves in which the mother is feeding the baby every 1–2 hours, night and day, to satisfy his needs—but by this time, exhaustion has set in. This is one of the main reasons why the milk supply decreases and women find they have to stop breast-feeding.

In the very early days I always advise a mother to assume that, if the baby is crying, then hunger is probably the main reason, and the baby should be fed. However, I do stress that if a baby is continually crying and unhappy, then you should look for reasons why the baby cannot last the three hours between feedings. Often the baby has not been latched on properly to the breast and, while he may appear to be constantly sucking for up to an hour, much of the time he is not actually drinking well. This is why mothers who are breast-feeding and finding that their baby is not going happily for 2–3 hours between feedings should always seek advice from a lactation consultant. Any healthy baby weighing more than 6 lbs. at birth should manage to go three hours between feedings—that is, three hours from the beginning of a feeding to the beginning of the next feeding (which ends up being only two hours between feedings). This will only happen if the baby receives enough breast milk to satisfy his needs.

Q **Do I really have to wake my newborn baby up to feed him? He wants to sleep all the time and I am tempted to leave him.**

A I do understand. It is a great temptation to catch up on other things during the daytime while your baby sleeps. But your baby will only be this sleepy for a few short weeks and he will then increasingly want to be awake, playing and having social time with you and others. He won't know the difference between day and night, and unless you gently guide him into a routine, you could end up with him wide awake and wanting to play games at 4 a.m. So, yes, I do stress the importance of waking the baby every 2–3 hours during the first week to ensure that the breasts are stimulated enough to increase the mother's milk production. Waking the baby every three hours throughout the day will ensure that the baby will more than likely wake only once in the night between midnight and 6 a.m. A mother who is well rested and relaxed will be much more likely to produce an abundant milk supply than a mother who is tired and stressed. In the long term, you will both benefit from establishing this pattern.

Q **Several friends and relations have said that it is cruel to wake a sleeping baby and that he will wake when he is ready to nurse. I am a very organized person and feel that following a routine would be best for both my baby and me, but I am frightened that I could do some sort of psychological or physical damage to my baby by waking him.**

A It is obvious that the people who say it is cruel to wake a sleeping baby to feed him have never had to care for very premature or sick babies, as I have. Waking these babies on a regular basis so they feed little and often was the only way to ensure their survival. Over the years, watching these babies grow up into young children, I have never seen any of them show signs of psychological or physical damage. I am convinced that there is a bigger risk of such damage to both baby and mother if a situation arises in which a baby is up and demanding to be fed every hour in the night. In the early days I advise feeding a baby little and often to establish breast-feeding. Sometimes this will involve waking him, but I advise that should a young baby demand feeding before three hours, then he must, of course, be fed. A pattern will quickly be established for both you and your baby from which you will both benefit.

Q The current advice is that parents should have their baby in the same room with them for all sleep periods during the first six months. I am concerned that my baby will not sleep well in our living room for naps and in the evening and that it will be difficult to get him used to sleeping in his nursery when he does reach six months. How easy is it to establish your routines while also adhering to the new guidelines?

A The majority of parents with whom I have worked have had their baby sleep with them in their room at night. The latest advice is that your baby should be put down for all his sleeping in the room you are in until he is six months old. This means that it will take more time to get him used to his nursery. However, getting your baby used to his own room sooner rather than later can help you avoid disrupting and unsettling him when he reaches six months. You can make the nursery a peaceful haven for him by using it for diaper changing, feeding and winding down or quiet playtime.

In terms of settling your baby to sleep in another room, try to keep things as calm and quiet as possible for him to help distinguish between "awake" time and time for sleeping. It is unlikely that you will have a crib in two places in your home; therefore, a bassinet with a proper, firm mattress would be an acceptable option. Follow the same guidelines for settling your baby in the bassinet as those given for settling him in a crib: place him in the bassinet with his feet at the bottom, and firmly tuck in any sheets and blankets. Putting the hood up during sleep times will help keep out the light and help your baby sleep better.

Last, remember that these recommendations are only for the first six months; after that you can start to settle your baby in his own room for naps and night-time sleep. (See Chapter Thirteen, Months Six to Nine, for advice on how to make the transition easier for him.)

Q Is it true that you say babies should not be cuddled? I keep reading that babies need lots of physical affection and attention in order for them to feel secure.

A I have always stressed the importance of physical contact and affection with your baby. However, I do say that parents should make sure that the cuddling and affection they give is to satisfy their baby's emotional needs before their own. And, crucially, there is a difference between cuddling your baby and cuddling him to sleep. If he gets used to the latter, it will create a dependence that you will have to break at some point— and it is much easier to get him used to settling himself to sleep when he is three weeks old than it will be when he is three months or three years old.

Q **While I would like a routine when my baby is born, I do not want to let him cry for long spells.**

A I would never advise that young babies should be left to cry for lengthy periods to get themselves to sleep. I do stress that some overtired babies will fight sleep, and they should be allowed a 5–10 minute "crying-down" period. They should *never* be left for any longer than this before they are checked again. I also stress that a baby should never be left to cry for even 2–3 minutes if there is any doubt that he could be hungry or need burping.

Some babies who have reached six months or a year and are waking several times a night because they have learned the wrong sleep associations, brought on by de-mand feeding or being rocked or cuddled to sleep, might need some form of sleep training.

Any form of sleep training is always a last resort to get an older baby to sleep during the night and should only be used once parents are absolutely sure that the baby is not waking because he is hungry. I also advise that before commencing sleep training you should take your baby to see the pediatrician to make sure there are no medical problems.

The whole aim of the CLB routines is to ensure that from the very beginning the baby's needs are being met so that he does not need to cry for any length of time. The guidelines I give are also to help mothers understand the different reasons why a baby might cry. If a baby is in a routine from a very early age, the mother will quickly learn to understand and even anticipate his needs. I have found that this results in the baby crying very seldom—around 5–10 minutes a day in my experience.

Q I have read that on your routines a baby should not be fed in the middle of the night once she reaches 12 weeks. Surely all babies are different and a baby should not be forced to go without food if she is hungry?

A Some babies, particularly breast-fed babies, may need to be fed once in the middle of the night until they are five or six months old. The majority of babies I have cared for would sleep through the night (i.e. from the late feeding until 6 to 7 a.m.) somewhere between eight and 12 weeks. The huge response that I've received from readers indicates that this is the average age at which babies forming routines will sleep for a longer period of time. Each baby, of course, is an individual, but if your baby does not sleep through the night until he is seven months old, neither you, nor I, nor your baby has "failed." My routines are there to help you begin to structure your days and nights, and perseverance will pay off when your baby is ready.

How quickly a baby sleeps through the night is very much determined by his weight and the amount of milk he is capable of drinking at each feeding during the day. Babies who are capable of drinking only small amounts would obviously need a feeding in the night for longer than a baby who is capable of drinking a larger amount at each feeding during the day. The aim of the CLB routines is not to push the baby through the night as quickly as possible or to deny the baby a feeding in the night if he genuinely needs one. It is to ensure that the baby receives most of his nutritional needs during the day so that when he is physically and mentally ready to go through the night he will automatically do so. The responses I have had, along with my many years of experience caring for babies, confirm that this approach works.

Q **I read a message from a mother in an online parenting chat room that she is very lonely and depressed following your routines as it leaves her no time to get out and do anything else.**

A I have always said that putting a young baby into a routine can be very demanding on the parents, particularly in the early weeks. However, by the time a baby is 2–3 months of age, a pattern has usually emerged in which the baby can stay awake for longer periods during the day and sleep for longer periods at night. In my experience of working with hundreds of mothers, their social outings were certainly restricted for the first 2–3 weeks, but after that, I cannot recall many mothers who did not manage to meet their friends most afternoons between 2 p.m. and 5 p.m. or for coffee in the mornings. Once you and your baby have gotten the hang of the routines, you can adapt them to suit you all better. The mothers I have worked with have felt that it is worth putting in the hard work at the beginning because the result is a contented baby who sleeps well at night and enjoys his social times during the day. A mother who has had a good night's sleep will be able to enjoy his days more, too!

I always advise mothers, in the early days, to try to ensure that at least every second day they arrange for a friend or relative to visit them so that they do not feel lonely or abandoned. I also stress the importance of a walk every day with the baby to get some fresh air.

Q **In your routines you tell mothers when to eat and drink. This strictness puts me off.**

A You can eat and drink whenever you like! In the early days mothers are often exhausted and put their own needs—even the basics such as eating and drinking—at the bottom of their list of priorities. Struggling with a newborn on your own can mean that you find yourself at lunchtime having only had a piece of toast and half a cup of tea. As a nursing mom, you need to eat plenty of food regularly and to drink plenty of water in order to produce enough milk for your baby and to keep up your own energy levels. I know that many people using my routines refer to my book several times a day so the hours suggested for breakfast and lunch and for drinking lots of water are a reminder not to neglect yourself—and they fit in with what your baby is doing, helping make it easier for you to care for yourself, too.

Q Why are your routines so rigid? Surely half an hour here or there won't make much difference?

A *The New Contented Little Baby Book* contains more than 10 different routines, taking you from week one of your baby's life right up to the end of his first year. They have been carefully compiled to allow for your baby growing and changing. As he goes through his first three months, he will gradually need less and less daytime sleep as he enjoys being awake and playing with you. He needs stimulation and fun during the day. He will need weaning at some point (current guidelines recommend exclusive breast-feeding for six months). His sleeping and eating needs are constantly changing throughout his first year of life. In my experience, adapting to your baby's changing needs is best done slowly and steadily. My routines are specific in order to help you to make those gradual changes. Once your baby is sleeping for 12 hours every night, you will feel a huge sense of relief, and he will be getting the long, deep sleep that he needs for healthy growth and development.

My routines are designed around babies' natural rhythms and they work. You do not have to stick rigidly to them, but half an hour discrepancy can end up disrupting the rest of your day and, possibly, your night. For example, if your day begins closer to 8 a.m. than 7 a.m., you will find your baby has a later nap at around 1 p.m. If he doesn't wake until after 3 p.m. you will find it difficult to get him to settle at 7 p.m., as he is unlikely to be sleepy by then. If the last feeding of the day is closer to 8 p.m., you could find as a result that he does not want his 10 p.m. feeding and will wake in the night. This is certainly not the end of the world occasionally but, over a period of time and as his nutritional needs change, you could find that he continues to wake at night, leaving you exhausted.

Q **I have been trying to follow your routines for four weeks but my baby is not anywhere close to fitting in with them. I feel like a failure and wonder if I should just give up and let her nurse and sleep whenever she wants.**

A It can be very difficult in the early days, and many parents understandably feel it would be easier on them if they let the baby decide what she wants to do. Bear in mind you are recovering from the birth; and looking after a baby, routine or not, is extremely hard work. My routines make sure the hard work is limited to as short a period as possible. Think how hard it would be if your baby were still waking in the night at nine months old. I can assure you it is worth persevering.

Don't necessarily expect instant contentment, but the result of sticking with the routines in the first weeks is a more enjoyable babyhood and toddlerhood for you and your child. When your baby does fit in, and she will very soon, the routines are there to help guide you and your baby into what represents the baby's natural patterns and rhythms. Remember that you are not "failing" if your baby doesn't fit in; just keep going, taking a day at a time. As every experienced parent and grandparent will be telling you—the first few months go very quickly.

Start each day at 7 a.m. and attempt to follow the day's routine, but if it has gone awry by lunchtime because your baby is wide awake at nap time and sleepy during the social times I suggest, don't panic. Keep repeating the same pattern of feedings and sleep every day as best you can, and your baby will pick it up very soon. If she is crying for food before I say she should be fed and you have tried distracting her or playing with her, then you must, of course, feed her. If you really cannot rouse her from a sleep when it's time to play, then leave her a bit longer and don't give yourself or her a hard time. Get up in the morning and try again without feeling you or your baby is getting it "wrong." I applaud mothers these days who are probably looking after their babies on their own during the days without the support of grandmas or aunties nearby. It's very hard work. You are not alone in going through the experience however, and you are certainly not a failure— it will get better!

Q **Why are you so strict about avoiding eye contact at the late feeding? I feel very cruel depriving my baby of cuddles and this close contact.**

A Please don't deprive your baby of cuddles! Nowhere do I suggest you should not cuddle your baby. On the contrary, a baby who is being held close to his mother, whether breast-fed or bottle-fed, will enjoy nursing and be ready to return to a contented sleep after he has been burped and settled down quietly. I suggest avoiding eye contact at the late and night feedings to help you show your baby gently that this is not playtime. Your cuddles can be very close, but overstimulating him during this winding-down time can cause him to become overtired and unable to settle well. He needs his sleep for his mental and physical development, and without it, he could become fretful, irritable and inconsolable. I feel it is better for the baby to be played with, sung to, shown interesting toys and books when he is wide awake and able to enjoy himself. Cuddling must be about your baby's needs and not just your own.

Q **Your routines are so strict. When can I enjoy my baby without worrying about what he should be doing next?**

A I sincerely hope that all parents enjoy their baby, from the first exciting day they come home from hospital, right through babyhood, toddlerhood and beyond. Every day is filled with opportunities for cuddling, playing, singing, reading, splashing in the bath, tickling toes while diaper changing and chatting to your baby. But it is beyond doubt that a contented baby is best able to appreciate and participate in these activities. My routines are there to support and help you find a structure to your days that will result in a contented baby. They are not for everyone, however, and if you feel stressed by following a routine then stop trying. My routines can help you avoid long-term problems, such as overtiredness due to overstimulation; sleep association in which a baby has to be rocked to sleep or driven round the block; or continual night waking that leaves you feeling exhausted each morning. Should any of these problems develop, you could turn to my book later for help.

Bonding evolves slowly over many weeks, and for many mothers without help or support, there can be— along with feelings of joy and love for a new baby— feelings of sheer exhaustion, failure and frustration. Nights of broken sleep do not help, and mothers often contact me because they feel guilty and resentful that they are not enjoying their baby. Weeks of sleep-deprivation caused by endless middle-of-the-night feeding are bound to hamper bonding and enjoyment of your baby. My routines are there to help you and your baby, not to cause stress, anxiety or feelings of inadequacy. A positive approach to them will help enormously.

Q **I have a toddler as well as a new baby to care for, and I cannot seem to get your routines to work around both of them.**

A This is an important point. Many mothers find that school schedules for older children mean that the nap times I suggest are not workable. If you used my routines with your first child, you will at least find the 7 a.m. start and 7 p.m. bedtime already established in your household. Your toddler may still take a lunchtime nap if he is less than three, and this can combine nicely with the baby's nap. You might even get an overlap of half an hour to yourself! I suggest that you concentrate on sticking to my suggested amounts of daytime sleep. So if you have to adapt your baby's daytime sleep around your toddler's routine, try not to let the baby exceed the recommended amount of daily sleep. Then bedtime will at least be guaranteed, and you can have an evening to rest and recover from caring for two young children.

3

Milk Feeding in the First Year

· · · · · ·

Successful feeding is of vital importance during the first year of your baby's life. It not only helps to lay the foundation for your baby's future health, but it also plays a huge part in how well your child sleeps. Breast milk is without a doubt the best food for your baby. I am proud to say that the majority of the mothers with whom I have worked managed successfully to breast-feed their babies until solids were introduced, and many for even longer than that. Of course, a few of my mothers only managed a few weeks, and others, for personal reasons, chose not to breast-feed at all. I hope that the advice in this book will help you successfully establish breast-feeding for your baby and, even if it does not appeal to you, that you will at least give it a try. Many mothers I have helped who hated breast-feeding their first baby because of the exhaustion of demand feeding found it to be a complete pleasure when following my CLB routines. If, for some reason, you have already given up or have chosen not to breast-feed, I still offer lots of advice on how to get bottle-feeding right.

The whole aim of my book is to help and support parents and, in particular, mothers, whom I know feel a huge amount of pressure these days about giving their baby the best start in life. Of course, breast milk is best, but the reality is that if formula were not a good substitute it would have been banned by the health authorities years ago. So if you have already given up breast-feeding or made a personal, informed choice not to, please do not feel guilty because of the disapproval of others. Ignore any negative comments, for example that you will not bond as closely with your baby. Speaking from personal experience, my own mother managed to breast-feed me for only about ten days, and no mother and daughter could have been closer than we were. Equally, I have friends who were breast-fed for nearly two years and cannot stand the sight of their mother!

However, I must stress that, contrary to advice from well-meaning family members, bottle-feeding does not necessarily guarantee you a more contented baby or make it easier to put him into a routine. Whether your baby is breast-fed or bottle-fed, it will still take time and perseverance to establish a routine, so please do not choose or change to formula thinking that you will have a more contented baby. A bottle-fed baby will need as much guidance and help into a routine as a breast-fed one; the only difference is that all the responsibility normally lies with the mother who is breast-feeding. For mothers who wish to breast-feed, the CLB routines will allow you to do so successfully and have a routine, with the bonus of your partner being able to give your baby a bottle as well.

. . . .

Why Breast-feeding Goes Wrong

The first thing that became obvious to me very early on when working with new mothers is that, while breast-feeding may be the most natural way to feed a newborn baby, for some mothers it does not come easily. Immediately after the birth, midwives encourage mothers to put their baby straight to the breast and guide them through the techniques of positioning and latching on the baby. For some mothers, their baby will latch on to the breast easily, feeding well and then drop off to sleep until the next feeding. For others the baby will fuss and fret, fight the breast or take several sucks before falling asleep. These problems are all very common in the early days. Mothers are now discharged from the hospital within 48 hours of giving birth and many are sent home without having grasped the basic latching-on techniques that are essential if breast-feeding is to be a success.

When I worked as a maternity nurse, I would often arrive at a family's home to find a mother with nipples that were so cracked and bleeding that she would be in tears every time she put the baby to her breast. In situations like this, breast-feeding and bonding get off to a very bad start for both mother and baby. The mother is in a lot of physical pain and also suffers mental agony, thinking she is not a good enough mother because her baby is not latching on properly. The baby gets stressed and cries a lot through hunger, because he is not nursing well enough. All of these problems, and many others associated with breast-feeding, could be avoided if more attention and help were given to the mother in the early days.

I believe passionately that the way to ensure more mothers breast-feed successfully is to give them help in the early days. While breast-feeding does come naturally to many mothers, it

. . . . .

does not come naturally to all, and we need to take this into account when we give advice.

How milk is produced and the composition of breast milk will also help you understand how the CLB feeding routines can and will work with breast-feeding, provided that you follow the advice on adjusting the routines to meet increased demand during growth spurts or at times when your baby has not taken a full feeding. The following brief summary gives an overview of how breast milk is produced. See resources at the back of the book for more in-depth information.

Milk Production

Milk Letdown Reflex

The hormones produced during your pregnancy help prepare your breasts for the production of milk. Once your baby is born and put to the breast to suck, a hormone called oxytocin is released from the pituitary gland at the base of your brain, which sends a "letdown" signal to the breast. The muscles supporting the milk glands contract and the milk is pushed down the 15 or 20 milk ducts as the baby sucks. Many women feel this as a slight tingling in their breasts and a contraction of their womb. These feelings normally disappear within a week or two. You may also experience a letdown when you hear your baby cry or if you think about him when you are apart. If you get tense or are very stressed, oxytocin is not released, making it difficult for your milk to let down. Therefore, it is essential for successful breast-feeding that you feel calm and relaxed. Preparing everything needed for a feeding in advance can help. Make sure you are sitting comfortably with your back straight and the baby well supported. Take time to position him onto the breast correctly. Pain caused by incorrect positioning also affects oxytocin being released, which in turn affects the letdown reflex.

Milk Composition

The first milk your breasts will produce is called colostrum. It is higher in protein and vitamins and lower in carbohydrate and fat than the mature milk that comes in between the third and fifth day. Colostrum also contains some of your antibodies, which will help your baby resist any infections you have had. Compared to the mature milk that soon follows, colostrum is much thicker and looks more yellow. By the second to third day, your breasts are producing a mixture of colostrum and mature milk. Then, somewhere between the third and fifth day, the breasts become engorged, and they will feel very hard, tender and often painful to the touch. This is a sign that the mature milk is fully in. The pain is caused not only by the milk coming in, but also by the enlargement of the milk glands and the increased blood supply to the breasts. When the milk comes in, it is essential to feed your baby little and often. Not only will it help stimulate a good milk supply, but also it will help relieve the pain of engorgement. During this time it may be difficult for your baby to latch onto the breast, and it may be necessary to express a little milk before feeding. This can be done by placing warm, wet cloths on the breasts and gently expressing a little milk by hand.

Mature milk looks very different from colostrum. It is thinner and looks slightly blue in color, and its composition also changes during the feeding. At the beginning of the feeding, your baby gets the fore milk, which is high in volume and low in fat. As the feeding progresses, your baby's sucking will slow down, and he will pause longer between sucks. This is a sign that he is reaching the hind milk. Although he only gets a small amount of hind milk, it is very important that he is left on the breast long enough to reach it. The hind milk will help your baby go longer between feedings. If you transfer him to the second breast before he has totally emptied the first breast, he will be more likely to get two lots of fore milk. This will end up leaving him feeling hungry again in a couple of hours. Another feeding of fore milk will quickly lead to your baby becoming very "colicky." While some babies do not get enough to eat from only one breast and need to be put on the second breast, always check that he has completely emptied the first breast before transferring him.

I find that at the end of the first week, by making sure babies are given around 25 minutes on the first breast, and offered the second breast for 5–15 minutes, I can be sure that they are getting the right balance of fore milk and hind milk. It also ensures that they are content to go between 3–4 hours before demanding their next feeding. If your baby is nursing from both breasts at each feeding, always remember to start the next feeding on the breast you last fed from, so that you can be certain each breast is totally emptied every second feeding.

In order to encourage a quick and easy letdown and to ensure that your baby gets the right balance of fore milk and hind milk, use the following guidelines:

❋ Make sure that you rest as much as possible between feedings and that you do not go too long between meals. Also, eat small, healthy snacks between meals.

❋ Prepare in advance everything needed for the feeding: a comfortable chair with arms and a straight back, and perhaps a footstool. Cushions to support both you and the baby, a drink of water and some soothing music will all help toward a relaxing, enjoyable experience for both of you.

* It is essential that you take your time to position the baby on the breast correctly; poor positioning leads to painful and often cracked, bleeding nipples.

* Always make sure your baby has completely emptied the first breast before putting him on the second. It is the small amount of high-fat hind milk that will help your baby go longer between feedings.

* Not all babies need the second breast in the early days. If your baby has totally emptied the first breast, burp him and change his diaper, then offer him the second breast. If he needs more he will take it. If not, start him off on that breast at the next feeding.

* If your baby does feed from the second breast, you should still start on that breast at the next feeding.

* Once the milk is in and you have built up the time your baby nurses from the breast, it is important that he is on the breast long enough to completely empty it and reach the hind milk. Some babies need up to 30 minutes to completely empty the breast. By gently squeezing your nipple between your thumb and fore-finger, you will be able to check if there is any milk still in the breast.

* Never, ever allow your baby to suck on an empty breast; this will only lead to very painful nipples.

. . . .

My Methods for Successful Breast-feeding

The key to successful breast-feeding is getting off to the right start, and as you will have already read, "little and often" after the birth is essential to helping establish a good milk supply. But putting the baby to the breast little and often will not guarantee you a good milk supply if your baby is not positioned on the breast properly. While in the hospital you might be guided by the nurses on how to latch your baby onto the breast. I strongly advise that you get help from an experienced lactation consultant. There are several organizations that will arrange for someone to visit you either in your home or at the office and spend time with you while you are nursing your baby to ensure that you are getting the positioning on the breast right. You might need several sessions to help overcome any problems that you may encounter in the early days.

I advise all my mothers to start on day one by offering five minutes each side every three hours, increasing the time by a few minutes each day until the milk comes in. The three hours is calculated from the beginning of one feeding to the beginning of the next feeding. Somewhere between the third and fifth day, your milk will be in, and you should have increased the baby's sucking time on the breast to 15–20 minutes. Many babies will now be getting enough milk from the first breast and be content to go three hours before needing to feed again.

However, if you find your baby is demanding food long before three hours have passed, he should, of course, be fed and also offered both breasts at each feeding if he still remains unsettled. It may take a sleepy baby 20–25 minutes to reach the very important hind milk (which is at least three times fattier than the fore milk) and to empty the breast. Other babies may

. . . . .

reach the hind milk much more quickly. Be guided by your baby as to how long he needs to feed well. If your baby nurses well, within the times I suggest, is happy and content between feedings and you are getting lots of wet diapers, he is obviously getting enough milk in the time he is on the breast.

POSITIONING THE BABY AT THE BREAST

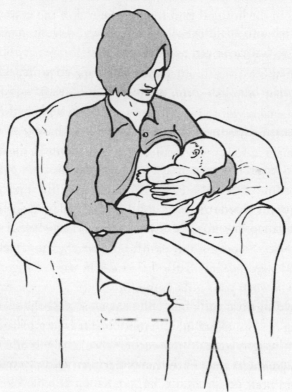

During the first few days, between 6 a.m. and midnight, wake your baby every three hours for short feedings. This will ensure that nursing gets off to the best possible start in time for when the milk comes in. Feeding your baby every three hours will help build up your milk supply much faster, and if he is fed enough during the day, your baby will be much more likely to go to sleep for longer periods between feedings in the night. It also avoids the mother becoming too exhausted, which, as I've said, is another major factor in breast-feeding going wrong. As with anything in life, success only comes from building a good foundation. All my mothers who establish every-three-hours feedings in the hospital find that by the end of the first week a pattern has emerged. Then, very quickly, they can adapt their baby's feeding pattern to my first routine.

The first breast-feeding routine (in Chapter Six, Weeks One to Two) not only helps you establish a good milk supply, but also will enable you to recognize all your baby's many different needs: hunger, tiredness, boredom and overstimulation.

The main reasons my breast-feeding methods are so successful:

✳ Feeding your baby every three hours in the first few days for shorter periods will gradually allow your nipples to get used to his sucking. This helps avoid the nipples becoming too painful or, even worse, cracked and bleeding. It will also help ease the pain of engorgement when your milk comes in.

✳ Feeding little and often will help avoid the baby spending hours sucking on an empty breast trying to satisfy his hunger, which often occurs when a baby is allowed to go longer than three hours between feedings in the first week.

✳ A newborn baby's tummy is tiny, and his needs can only be satisfied by feeding little and often. If you nurse your baby every three hours between 6 a.m. and midnight, the "feeding all night syndrome" should never occur. Even a very small baby is capable of going one longer spell in between feedings. Following my advice ensures that this will happen at night and not during the day.

* Successful breast-feeding can only be achieved if a mother feels relaxed and comfortable. This is impossible if, having just given birth, you become exhausted from being awake and nursing your baby all night.

* Newborn babies do not know the difference between day and night. Your baby will learn the difference much sooner if you differentiate between daytime feedings and nighttime feedings and do not allow him to sleep for long spells between feedings from 7 a.m. to 7 p.m.

Expressing/Pumping

I believe that expressing milk in the early days plays a huge part in determining how successful a mother will be in breast-feeding while following a routine. I am convinced that one of the main reasons the majority of my mothers have the success that they do is because I encourage the use of an electric breast pump in the first few weeks.

The simple reason is that breast milk is produced on a supply and demand basis. During the very early days, most babies will empty the first breast and some may take a small amount from the second breast. Very few will empty both breasts at this stage. By the end of the second week, the milk production balances out and most mothers are producing exactly the amount their baby is demanding. Some time during the third and fourth week, the baby goes through a growth spurt and demands more milk. This is where a problem often sets in.

In order to meet the increased demand for more food, you would more than likely have to go back to feeding every two or three hours and often twice in the night. This pattern is repeated each time the baby goes through a growth spurt and often results in the baby being continually fed just before sleep time. This creates the problem of the wrong sleep association, making it even more difficult to get the baby back into the routine.

Mothers who express the extra milk they produce in the very early days will always be producing more than their baby needs. When their baby goes through a growth spurt, the routine stays intact, because simply expressing less milk at the early-morning feedings can immediately satisfy any increased appetite.

Expressing from the very early days can also avoid the problem of a low milk supply. However, if your baby is more than one month old and you already have the problem of a low milk supply, by following my plan for increasing your milk supply (see Common Feeding Problems in Chapter Sixteen), you should see a big improvement within six days. For babies less than one month old, following the expressing times laid out in the routines should be enough to increase your supply.

If you decided at some point between one and four weeks to introduce a bottle of either expressed milk or formula at the late feeding, you will be able to hand over feeding responsibility to someone else. This means you can get to bed early. I advise that you express some milk at this time or that you are feeding the baby. If the baby takes a bottle, then you can express between 9:30 p.m. and 10 p.m. and then go to bed. Expressing milk at this time is important to keep the supply going and ensure you have plenty for the middle-of-the-night feeding.

If you have previously experienced difficulties with expressing, do not be disheartened. Expressing at the time suggested in my routines or the plan in Chapter Sixteen, Problem Solving in the First Year, along with the following guidelines, should help:

٭ The best time to express is in the morning as the breasts are usually fuller. Expressing will also be easier if done at the beginning of a feeding. Express one breast just before feeding your baby, or feed your baby from one breast, then express from the second breast before offering him the remainder of his feeding. Some mothers actually find that expressing is easier when done while they are feeding the baby on the other breast. It is also important to note that expressing at the beginning of a feeding allows slightly longer for that breast to make more milk for the next feeding.

In my routines I suggest that the mother expresses at 6:45 a.m.; however, if you are producing a lot of milk and can't face the early-morning slot, you could move the expressing of the second breast to around 7:30 a.m. after the baby has fed from the first breast. A mother who is concerned about her milk supply or who is following the plan for increasing the milk (see Common Feeding Problems) should try to stick to the recommended times.

٭ In the early days, you will need to allow at least 15 minutes to express 2–3 oz. at the morning feedings, and up to 30 minutes at the evening. Keep expressing times quiet and relaxed. The more you practice, the easier it will become. I usually find that, by the end of the first month, the majority of my mothers can easily express 2–3 oz. within ten minutes at the 9:30 p.m. expressing when using a double electric breast pump.

٭ An electric breast pump, the type used in hospitals, is by far the best way to express milk in the early days.

The suction of these machines is designed to simulate a baby's sucking rhythm, encouraging the milk flow. If you are expressing both breasts at 9:30 p.m., it is also worthwhile investing in an attachment that enables both breasts to be expressed at once, therefore reducing the time spent expressing.

* Sometimes, the letdown is slower in the evening when the breasts are producing less milk. A relaxing warm bath or shower will often encourage the milk to flow more easily. Also, gently massaging the breasts before and during expressing will help.

* Some mothers find that it is helpful to set up a regular way to relax, whether it is reading a book or watching a favorite television program or something else. Experiment with different approaches to see which one works best for you.

As you proceed through the routines, you will see that I advise which expressing times to drop. Essentially, you will cut back on expressing as your milk supply becomes firmly established. By three months you will only be expressing for the late feeding and, some time between four and six months, you can cut out this final expressing. Once your milk supply is reliably established to suit your baby you can be flexible with the 9:30 p.m. expressing. If you don't do it some nights, it won't be a problem. The reason I advise continuing to express into the fourth and fifth month is so you will have extra milk to give your baby as he shows signs of needing to be weaned. If you decide to wean before six months (after advice from a health professional) you can stop expressing right away.

Breast-feeding and Returning to Work

If you are planning to return to work and would like to continue to breast-feed, it is important that you make sure that you have established a good milk supply, especially if you want your baby to have expressed breast milk during the day. A three-month-old baby will need two feedings of approximately 7–8 oz. each of expressed milk if you are out between 9 a.m. and 5 p.m. As your baby will most likely be emptying both breasts at the 7 a.m. and 6 p.m. feedings, you will need to express most of the milk for the feedings to be given in your absence during the working day or between 9 p.m. and 10 p.m. in the evening.

You should fit in two expressing sessions at around 10 a.m. and 2:30 p.m. If you express any later than this, it is possible that your breasts will not produce enough for the 6 p.m. feeding, especially if you are in a hurry to get home.

The following guidelines give suggestions on how to incorporate working and breast-feeding:

* The longer you can spend at home establishing a milk supply, the easier it will be to maintain it once you return to work.
* Expressing from the beginning of the second week at the times suggested will enable you to build up a good stock of breast milk in your freezer.
* Introducing a bottle of expressed milk at the late feeding by the second week will ensure that there will not be a problem of your baby not taking the bottle when you return to work.
* Check with your employer well in advance of returning to work to ensure that a quiet place will be available

where you can express. Also check that you will be allowed to store the expressed milk in the refrigerator.

✳ Make sure that the nursery, or your child-care provider, is familiar with the storage and handling of breast milk, and how to defrost it.

✳ Establish the combined breast-and-bottle routine that you will be using for your baby at least two weeks in advance of your return to work. This will allow you plenty of time to sort out any difficulties that may arise.

✳ Once you return to work, it is essential that you pay particular attention to your diet and that you rest well in the evening. I suggest you continue expressing at 9:30 p.m. to ensure that you maintain a good milk supply.

✳ Also, make sure that you keep a good supply of breast pads at work, and a spare shirt or top!

Weaning Your Baby from the Breast to the Bottle

However long you have breast-fed, it is important to plan the transition from breast-feeding to bottle-feeding properly. When deciding how long you intend to breast-feed your baby, you should take into consideration that once you have established a good milk supply, you must allow approximately a week to drop each feeding. For example, it can take six weeks to establish a good milk supply, and if you decide to give up breast-feeding, you should allow, at the very least, a further five weeks to drop all breast-feeding and establish bottle-feeding. This information is very important for mothers who are planning to continue working. If you give up breast-feeding before you have established a good milk supply, you should still allow enough time for your baby to get used to feeding from the bottle. Some babies can get very upset if they suddenly lose the pleasure and comfort they get from breast-feeding.

For a mother who has breast-fed for less than a month, I generally advise waiting a period of 3–4 days before dropping each feeding. For a mother who has been breast-feeding longer than a month, it is best to allow 5–7 days before dropping each feeding. Assuming that the baby is already being bottle-fed at the late feeding, the next breast-feed to drop should be at 11 a.m. The best way to do this is gradually to reduce the length of time the baby nurses from the breast by five minutes each day and top up with formula. Once your baby is taking a full bottle-feeding, the breast-feeding can be dropped. If you plan the weaning carefully from the breast to formula, your baby will have time to adjust to the bottle, and you avoid the risk of developing mastitis. This can happen if the milk ducts become blocked due to engorgement, a common problem among mothers who instantly drop a feeding.

I suggest that you continue to express at 9:30 p.m. throughout the weaning process. The amount of milk expressed will be an indicator of how quickly your milk supply is going down.

Some mothers find that once they are down to two breast-feedings a day, their milk reduces very rapidly. The signs to watch out for: your baby being irritable and unsettled after nursing or wanting a feeding long before it is normally due. If your baby shows either of these signs, he should be topped up immediately after the breast-feeding with 1–2 oz. of expressed milk or formula. This will ensure that his sleeping pattern does not go wrong due to hunger.

The chart below is a guideline for which feedings to drop first. Each stage represents the period before you drop each feeding—either 3–4 days or 5–7 days, depending upon how long you have been breast-feeding.

TIME OF FEEDINGS	7 A.M.	11 A.M.	2:30 P.M.	6:30 P.M.	10 P.M.
Stage one	Breast	Formula`	Breast	Breast	Express*
Stage two	Breast	Formula	Formula	Breast	Express
Stage three	Breast	Formula	Formula	Formula	Express
Stage four	Breast	Formula	Formula	Formula	
Stage five	Formula	Formula	Formula	Formula	

*I recommend that mothers should continue to express for the late feeding (provided the baby is taking his bottle from his father or another helper) until the baby is 3–4 months old. This helps maintain a good milk supply, and can be used as an approximate gauge of how much milk you are producing. I find that a mother will usually produce overnight roughly twice the amount she has expressed. When you reach stage three of the weaning process, the 9:30 p.m. expressing should be dropped gradually, reducing the expressing time by three minutes each night. Once you are only expressing 2 oz. and going comfortably through the night, the expressing can be dropped altogether. When the last breast-feed has been dropped, care should be taken not to stimulate the breasts. Sitting in a warm bath with the water covering the breasts helps to get rid of any small amount of milk remaining in the breasts without stimulating them to make more.

. . . .

Bottle-feeding

If you have decided to bottle-feed, the same routines as for breast-feeding should be followed. The only difference is that you may find your baby is happy to go longer than three hours after the 7 a.m. feeding; otherwise the timing is exactly the same. When a feeding is being split—i.e. one breast before the bath and one after—the same pattern applies to bottle-feeding. I would normally make two separate smaller bottles for this time.

How Much and How Often?

Health authorities advise that a baby less than four months would need 2½ oz. of milk for each pound of his body weight; a baby weighing around 7 lbs. would need approximately 18 oz.

. . . . .

a day. This is only a guideline; hungrier babies may need an extra ounce at some feedings. If your baby is one of these, ensure that you structure your feedings so he is taking the bigger feedings at the right times; i.e., 7 a.m., 10:30 a.m. or 10:30 p.m. If you allow him to get into the habit of having bigger feedings in the middle of the night, it would eventually have the domino effect of him not being so hungry when he wakes in the morning. A vicious circle emerges in which he needs to feed in the night because he does not get enough during the day.

The same guidelines apply for breast-feeding: Aim to get the baby to take most of his daily milk requirements between 7 a.m. and 11 p.m. This way he will only need a small feeding in the middle of the night and will eventually drop it altogether.

The chart below is an example of the feeding pattern of one of my babies during his first month. He weighed 7 lbs. at birth and, with a weekly gain of 6–8 oz., reached just more than 9 lbs. when he was one month old. By structuring the feedings with the right ones at the right times, he was well on the way to dropping his middle-of-the-night feeding, and at six weeks, he was sleeping through to 6:30 a.m.

TIMES	7 A.M.	10–10:30 A.M.	2–2:30 P.M.	5 P.M.	6:15 P.M.	10–11 P.M.	2–3 A.M.	TOTAL
Week 1	(3 oz.)	(3 oz.)	(3 oz.)	(2 oz.)	(2 oz.)	(3 oz.)	(3 oz.)	(19 oz.)
Week 2	(3 oz.)	(4 oz.)	(3 oz.)	(3 oz.)	(2 oz.)	(4 oz.)	(2 oz.)	(21 oz.)
Week 3	(4 oz.)	(4 oz.)	(3 oz.)	(3 oz.)	(3 oz.)	(4 oz.)	(3 oz.)	(24 oz.)
Week 4	(5 oz.)	(4 oz.)	(4 oz.)	(3 oz.)	(3 oz.)	(5 oz.)	(2 oz.)	(26 oz.)

N.B. These daily amounts of milk were calculated to suit that particular baby's needs. Remember to adjust the quantities of milk to suit your own baby's needs, but still follow the feeding times shown. During growth spurts make sure that the 7 a.m., 10–10:30 a.m. and 10–11 p.m. feedings are the first to be increased.

. . . .

Establishing Bottle-feeding

When your baby is born, the hospital may provide you with ready-made formula. You may be given a choice of a number of different commercial brands. There is very little difference among them in their composition. The bottles of formula will come with prepacked sterilized nipples, which are used once and then thrown away. Unless the jars have been stored in the fridge, they do not need to be heated; they can be given at room temperature. However, if for some reason you do decide to heat the formula, do so by using either an electric bottle-warmer or by standing the bottle in a pan of boiling water.

Never heat the formula in a microwave, as the heat may not be evenly distributed and you could end up scalding your baby's mouth. Whichever form of heating you use, always test the temperature before giving the bottle to your baby. Shaking a few drops on the inside of your wrist can do this; it should feel lukewarm, never hot. Once milk is heated, it should never be reheated, as this very rapidly increases the bacteria levels in the milk, which is one of the main causes of upset tummies in formula-fed babies.

The advice given in the hospital for formula-fed babies seems to be much the same as for breast-fed babies: Feeding on demand whenever the baby wants and however much he wants. While you do not have the problem of establishing a milk supply as in breast-feeding, many of the other problems are likely to occur. A bottle-fed baby weighing 7 lbs. or more at birth could go straight on to the one- to two-week routine, for example. A smaller baby might not manage to last quite as long between feedings and need to be fed closer to every three hours.

Ready-made formula is incredibly expensive to use all the

. . . . .

time; most parents only use it on outings or in emergencies. Before leaving the hospital, arrange for someone to buy at least two large cans of powdered formula milk of the same brand as the ready-made milk to which your baby has already been introduced at the hospital. Make sure it is appropriate for newborns.

Once home, you will get into a routine of making up bottles. The World Health Organization recommends mixing formula with water that is at least 158 degrees. According to the Food and Drug Administration, boiling water for at least one minute is sufficient to sterilize it for a newborn. Allow it to cool to body temperature before giving it to your baby. If you need to make feedings in advance, for example for a nighttime feeding or to take on an outing, put some boiled water into a sterilized vacuum flask. When away from home, take the flask, together with the right amount of powder in a cleaned, sterilized and dry plastic container and the cleaned, sterilized bottle. Make the feeding and cool the bottle before feeding it to your baby. You may also wish to buy some cartons of ready-made formula to be used occasionally in emergencies, although these are a more expensive option.

Hygiene and Sterilization

The utmost attention must be paid to hygiene: the sterilizing of all your baby's feeding equipment and the preparation and storing of his formula milk.

The area where you sterilize and prepare your baby's formula should be kept spotless, washed with hot, soapy water and wiped daily with antibacterial cleaner.

The guidelines listed, if followed to the letter, will reduce the risk of germs, which are so often the cause of stomach upsets in infants:

* Surfaces should be washed down thoroughly every day, as described previously.
* After each feeding, the bottle and nipple should be rinsed thoroughly, using cold water, and put aside in a bowl ready for washing and sterilizing.
* Get into the habit of sterilizing once a day.
* Hands should always be washed thoroughly with antibacterial soap under warm running water and then dried with paper towels.
* Boil water on the stove and then use it to fill the bowl of dirty bottles with hot, soapy water. Using a long-handled bottlebrush, carefully scrub all the bottles, rims, caps and nipples inside and out. Particular attention should be given to the necks and rims. Carefully rinse everything under hot, running water. Wash and rinse the bowl thoroughly, then place all the equipment in the bowl under the running hot water. This is to check that everything is thoroughly rinsed—the water should run clear.
* The sterilizer should be rinsed out every day and the removable parts checked and, if necessary, washed and rinsed. The bottles and nipples should then be packed into the sterilizer following the manufacturer's instructions.

Giving the Feeding

Prepare everything in advance: chair, cushions, bib and burp cloth. As with breast-feeding, it is important that you are sitting comfortably, and in the early days I advise all mothers to support the arm in which they are holding the baby with a pillow, which enables you to keep the baby on a slight slope with his back straight. By holding the baby as shown in diagram A on page 83, you will lessen the likelihood of your baby getting air trapped in his tummy, which he might if fed as shown in diagram B. Before you start to feed the baby, loosen and screw the nipple back on; it should be very slightly loose. If it is screwed on too tightly it will not allow air into the bottle, and your baby will end up sucking and not getting any milk.

Check also that the milk is not too hot; it should be just slightly warm. If you get your baby used to very warm milk, you will find that, as the feeding progresses and the milk gets cool, he will refuse to feed. As it is dangerous to reheat the milk or keep it standing in hot water for any length of time, you could end up having to make two bottles for every feeding.

Once your baby is feeding, make sure that the bottle is kept tilted up far enough to ensure that the nipple is always filled with milk, to prevent your baby from taking in too much air. Allow your baby to drink as much as he wants before stopping to burp him. If you burp him before he is ready, he will only become very cranky and upset.

Some babies will take most of their feeding, burp and then want a break of 10–15 minutes before finishing the remainder of the milk. In the early days—allowing for a break midway—it can take up to 40 minutes to give the bottle. Once your baby is 6–8 weeks old, he will most likely finish feeding in about 20 minutes.

If you find your baby is taking a very long time to feed, or keeps falling asleep halfway through, it could be because the hole in the nipple is too small. I find that many of my babies have to go straight on to a medium-flow nipple as the slow-flow one is too slow.

Occasionally, there are babies who will drink a full feeding in 10–15 minutes and look for more. These babies are often referred to as "hungrier babies"; the reality is that these babies are usually "sucky" babies, not hungrier ones. Because they have such a strong suck, they are able to finish the bottle very quickly. Sucking is not only a means of feeding to a baby, but also in the early days, one of his natural pleasures. If your baby is taking the required amount of formula at each feeding very quickly and looking for more, it may be worth trying a nipple with a smaller hole. Offering him a pacifier after feedings may also help satisfy his "sucking needs."

It is very easy for bottle-fed babies to gain weight too quickly if they are allowed to have feedings well in excess of the amounts recommended for their weight. While a few ounces a day should not create a problem, a baby who is overeating, and regularly putting on more than 8 oz. each week, will eventually become overweight and reach a stage at which milk alone is not enough to satisfy his hunger. If this happens before the recommended age for giving solids, it can create a real problem.

For establishing successful bottle-feeding, the following guidelines should be observed:

* Before beginning the feeding, check that the ring holding the nipple and the bottle together is very slightly loose; if it is too tight, it will restrict the flow of the milk.
* Check that the milk is the right temperature; it should be lukewarm, not hot.
* To avoid gas problems, which are very common among formula-fed babies, always make sure that you are comfortable and holding your baby correctly before beginning the feeding.
* Some very young babies need a break in the middle of the feeding. Allow up to 40 minutes for your baby to take a full feeding.

POSITIONING OF YOUR BABY WHILE BOTTLE-FEEDING

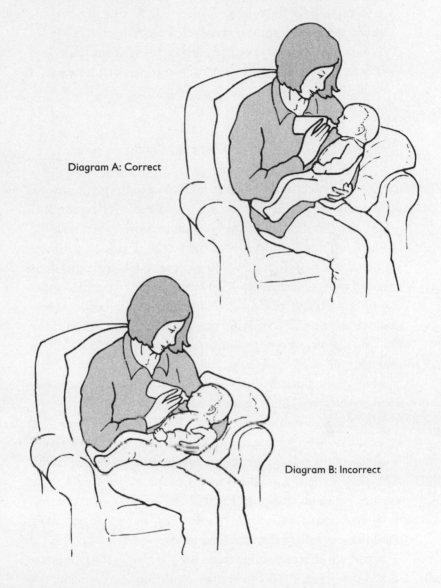

Diagram A: Correct

Diagram B: Incorrect

✳ If you find you are always having to wake your baby for the 7 a.m. feeding, only to find he is not so hungry, then cut back the middle-of-the-night feeding by 1 oz.

✳ During growth spurts, make sure you follow the guidelines in Chapter Four, Understanding Your Baby's Sleep. This will avoid your baby cutting back, or even dropping, the wrong feedings first.

. . . .

Formula: Overfeeding

Unlike the breast-fed baby, the most common problem in the early days with formula-fed babies is overfeeding. The reason I believe this can happen with some babies is that they take the bottle of formula so quickly that their natural sucking instincts are not satisfied and they end up screaming when the bottle is removed from their mouth. Many mothers interpret this cry as one of hunger and end up giving them another bottle of formula. A pattern of overfeeding can quickly emerge, resulting in the baby gaining huge amounts of weight each week. If this problem is allowed to continue, the baby quickly reaches a stage at which milk alone will not satisfy his appetite, yet he is too young to be given solids (less than six months).

While it is normal for some babies to need an additional 1 oz. at some feedings, special attention should be given if a baby is taking in excess of 5 oz. every day, and is regularly gaining more than 8 oz. each week. When my formula-fed babies show signs of being particularly "sucky," I have found that offering some cool boiled water between feedings and a pacifier afterward helps to satisfy their sucking needs.

If you are concerned that your baby is overfeeding, it is essential that you discuss the problem with your pediatrician.

. . . . .

Your Questions Answered

Q I have very small breasts and am worried that I may not be able to produce enough milk to satisfy my baby's needs.

A Breast size is totally irrelevant when it comes to producing breast milk. Each breast, regardless of shape or size, has 15–20 ducts, each duct with its own cluster of milk-making cells. Milk is made within these cells and pushed down the ducts when the baby sucks.

✳ During the early days, make sure your baby is put to the breast frequently. Most babies need a minimum of eight feedings a day to help stimulate the breasts and establish a good milk supply.

✳ Always make sure that your baby totally empties the first breast before putting him on the second breast. This signals the breast to make more milk and also ensures that your baby gets the important hind milk.

Q My friend was in agony when her milk came in. Is there anything I can do to help relieve the pain of engorgement?

A Put your baby to the breast often and do not let him go longer than three hours during the day or 4–5 hours at night between feedings.

✳ A warm bath or warm, wet cloths placed on the breasts before a feeding will help the milk flow and, if need be, gently expressing a little milk by hand will make it easier for the baby to latch on.

* Damp cloths chilled in the fridge and placed on the breasts after a feeding will help constrict the blood vessels and reduce the swelling.

* Wear a well-fitting nursing bra that supports your breasts. Make sure that it is not too tight under the arms and does not flatten your nipples.

Q **Many of my friends had to give up breast-feeding because it was so painful.**

A The main reason women experience pain in the early days is because the baby is not positioned on the breast correctly. The baby ends up chewing on the end of the nipple, causing much pain for the mother, more often than not resulting in cracked, bleeding nipples and a poor feeding for the baby. A pattern soon emerges of the baby needing to feed again very quickly, giving him even more opportunity to damage the nipples.

* Make sure that you always hold your baby with his tummy to your tummy and that his mouth is open wide enough for him to take all of the nipple and as much of the areola as he can manage into his mouth. Apart from ensuring that your baby is well positioned, it is important that you are sitting comfortably. The ideal chair should have a straight back, preferably with arms so that you can position a cushion to support the arm in which you are holding the baby. If you do not support your arm, it will be much more difficult to position and support your

baby properly. This can cause him to pull on the breast, which will be painful for you.

Q **I have a three-week-old baby and am getting very concerned over the conflicting advice. Some people say give both breasts at each feeding; others say one is enough.**

A Be guided by your baby. If he nurses from one breast, is content to go 3–4 hours between feedings, and is gaining weight steadily each week, one breast is obviously enough.

* If he is looking for food after two hours, or is waking in the night more than once, it would be advisable to offer him the second breast. You may find he only needs the second breast later in the day when your milk supply is at its lowest.

* Always check that the first breast is completely empty before putting him on the second. This can be done by gently squeezing the area around the nipple between your thumb and forefinger.

Q **Do I need to avoid certain foods while breast-feeding?**

A You should continue with the same varied, healthy diet that you followed throughout your pregnancy. In addition, you should include small healthy snacks between meals to help keep your energy level up and take in extra calcium. The National Academy of Sciences recommends that women who are pregnant or breast-feeding consume 1,000 mg of calcium each day.

* * * * *

✳ Ensure that you eat at least 6 oz. of either poultry, lean meat or fish each day. Vegetarians should eat the equivalent in beans, peas and rice, etc. I have noticed that on the days when some of my breast-feeding mothers did not eat enough protein, their babies were much more unsettled.

✳ Some research points to dairy products as the cause of colic in certain babies. If you find your baby develops colic, it may be wise to discuss with your pediatrician how to monitor your dairy intake.

✳ Alcohol, artificial sweeteners and caffeine should be avoided. Remember that caffeine is found not only in coffee, but also in tea, soft drinks and chocolate. I have found all of these things can upset most babies.

✳ Strawberries, tomatoes, mushrooms, onions and fruit juice, if taken in large quantities, have left many of my babies very irritable. While I do not suggest cutting all of these from your diet, I do suggest that you take note of any food or drink consumed 12–16 hours before your baby began showing signs of a stomachache, explosive bowel movements, excessive gas and crying fits.

✳ Although it is advisable to avoid alcohol, especially spirits, while breast-feeding, some experts advise that a small glass of wine or beer can be beneficial to a mother who is finding it hard to unwind in the evening.

Q **My two-week-old baby wakes yelling to be fed, only to fall asleep after five minutes on the breast. He then demands to be fed two hours later, leaving me absolutely exhausted.**

⋆ ⋆ ⋆ ⋆ ⋆

A   Always make sure your baby is fully awake before you attempt to feed him. Unwrap him in the crib, take his legs out of his nightclothes and allow the cool air to get to his skin, giving him time to wake by himself. Then you can start to feed him.

* It is very important that sleepy babies are kept cool while feeding. He should not be overdressed and the room should not be too warm. Have a play mat next to you on the floor, and the minute he gets sleepy, put him on it. If necessary, remove his onesie, as this will encourage him to stretch and kick. Within a few minutes he will probably protest about being put down, so pick him up and give him a few more minutes on the same breast. Often this procedure has to be repeated two or three times. Once he has had 20 minutes on the first breast, burp him well and change his diaper. He can then be put back on the first breast if he has not emptied it or transferred to the second.

* If possible, get your partner to do the late feeding with a bottle. This way, you will at least manage to get an uninterrupted few hours' sleep for one part of the night.

Q   My son is 16 weeks old. Over the last two weeks, he has become increasingly difficult to nurse. He dropped the middle-of-the-night feeding at around 11 weeks old yet, despite not feeding after the late feeding, he is fairly disinterested in his 7 a.m. feeding, taking as little as 2 oz. He then cries on and off until I feed him at 11 a.m. When I feed him earlier than 11 a.m., he then does not sleep well at

lunchtime, waking after an hour looking to nurse. When I feed him then, it upsets the feeding schedule for the rest of the afternoon.

A   To get your son more interested in his 7 a.m. feeding, try cutting back on his late feeding. Although he will need a small feeding at this time, probably until he is weaned onto solids, try reducing it gradually until you get it down to 3–4 oz.

∗ Until he is feeding better at 7 a.m., you will have to feed him earlier than 11 a.m., possibly by 10:15 a.m., but I would suggest that you top him up around 11:15/11:30 a.m. to ensure that he has taken enough milk so he sleeps well at his lunchtime nap.

∗ You may also find that when he goes through a growth spurt he starts to take his morning bottle much more quickly and may even start waking earlier, wanting to nurse. When this happens I suggest that you go back to giving him more at the late feeding to ensure he gets through to 7 a.m. You may have to do this for a week or so, and perhaps even continue with a larger feeding until he is weaned. However, if he starts to get fussy about the morning feeding again, you would then have to cut back on the late feeding once more.

4

Understanding Your Baby's Sleep

· · · · · ·

Sleep is probably the most misunderstood and confus-
ing aspect of parenthood. The misconception is that
for the first few weeks all an infant will do is feed and sleep.
While many do, there are more than 126 sleep clinics in
the United Kingdom for babies and children, which is
proof that a great many do not. If your newborn or young
baby is one of the latter—tense, cranky and difficult to
settle—please take heart, as this need not be a reflection of
your baby's future sleep habits.

The majority of babies that I have helped care for usually
started to sleep until 6–7 a.m. somewhere between 8 and
12 weeks. A few slept through before that age, while some
still needed to be fed in the night for much longer. As I do
not know your baby personally, I cannot give you a specific
answer as to when he will sleep through, as many factors
will dictate that. For example, if your baby was born pre-
maturely or you did not start following the routines until

he was several weeks old, then obviously he may take longer to sleep through the night.

The important thing to remember is that what you are trying to achieve in the early days is a regular sleeping pattern. Your baby will settle well in the evening, nurse and settle again after the late feeding, wake just once in the night for a feeding and go back to sleep quickly until 6–7 a.m.

The aim of the routines is to achieve this without causing distress to you or your baby; it is not about pushing your baby through the night at the earliest possible age without feeding him. By following the guidelines I have laid out in this book, and adjusting the routines to suit your baby's own particular needs, he will sleep the longest spell at night as soon as he is physically and mentally capable of doing so.

The key to achieving this is to be patient and consistent and allow time for my routines to become established. Once they are, you can avoid the agony of months of sleepless nights that so many parents go through. It has worked for hundreds of thousands of babies and their parents, so it can work for you!

If you want your baby to sleep through the night from an early age and ensure a long-term healthy sleep pattern, the golden rules are **to establish the right associations and to structure your baby's feedings from the day you arrive home from the hospital.** The advice given in many of the baby books, and by some hospital staff, is that newborn babies should feed on demand for as often and for as long as they need. You will be told to accept that your baby's erratic sleeping and feeding patterns are normal and that things will improve by three months of age. Since the publication of my first book in 1999, I have received countless phone calls, e-mails and letters from distraught mothers whose infants, aged anywhere between three months and three years, have serious sleep and feeding problems. This continually disproves the theory that babies will put themselves into a routine by three months. Even if a baby does do this, it is unlikely to be a routine that fits neatly with the rest of the family's schedule.

While some experts agree that some babies are capable of sleeping through the night by three months, they do not stress the importance of guiding the baby toward this goal. The innocent and weary parent believes in and hopes for a miraculous improvement at three months, but this is unlikely to happen if her baby has not learned the difference between day and night and naps and the long sleep and if the parent has not learned how to structure feedings from day one. Ensuring that your baby feeds little and often during the day is essential if you want to avoid his waking genuinely hungry every couple of hours during the night.

When I ran my consultancy service for new parents I would, on a daily basis, receive desperate calls from the maternity wards. The cry for help was nearly always the same. The baby is feeding for up to an hour at a time, usually every two hours from 6 p.m. until 5 a.m. The mother is often exhausted and starting to suffer from cracked nipples.

When I ask what the baby is like during the day the usual reply is: "He's ever so good during the day; he will feed, then go four hours or longer."

It continues to baffle me that such contradictory advice is still being given to new parents. They are told that it is normal for a newborn baby to need to feed as much as 8–12 times a day, but they should then allow the baby to sleep hours between daytime feedings. It is hardly surprising that a baby who has had only four or even fewer feedings between 6 a.m. and 6 p.m. is going to wake many times in the night to satisfy his daily needs. This is one of the main reasons that I am opposed to the advice that babies should be demand fed. It does not take into account that many babies do not demand to be fed in the early days.

Sleep and Demand Feeding

The term *demand feeding* is used time and time again, misleading a mother into believing that any sort of routine in the early days could deny her baby nutritionally and, according to some experts, emotionally. While I would totally agree that the old-fashioned every-four-hours-feeding routine, whether breast or bottle, is not natural to newborn babies, I feel the term *feeding on demand* is used too loosely.

The pattern for sleepless nights is unfortunately often set before mother and baby leave the hospital. Because the baby has been allowed to sleep for long spells between feedings during the day, he genuinely needs to nurse on and off all evening and every couple of hours in the night. A vicious circle soon emerges in which the baby is sleeping for most of the day because he has been awake most of the night. Many experts encourage this type of sleeping-and-feeding pattern as they believe that the baby should take the lead when feeding is concerned. Hence the terms *baby-led feeding* or *demand feeding*. Some experts even go as far as to say that it is "damaging" to wake a sleeping baby and take a very hostile view of my advice to do so. It was my experience of working with many sets of twins and premature babies that helped me to realize this was complete nonsense. I observed that when I went to care for these babies, the hospital staff had already implemented a feeding routine. Because the lives of these tiny, sleepy babies depended upon being fed little and often, they would not have dared take the risk of allowing them to go long spells between feedings. This experience went a long way in helping me develop the CLB routines. Contrary to what some people imply, the routines are not about denying the baby food, but about ensuring that they are fed enough. As I have already mentioned, I have had personal experience of caring for infants who nearly lost their lives due to dehydration because they were not demanding to be fed enough. This further convinced me that demand-feeding puts an infant at much more risk than if he is woken at regular intervals to eat.

Because breast milk is produced on a supply-and-demand basis—i.e. the breasts make the amount of milk that the baby demands—within a few weeks the demand-fed baby often starts to demand to be fed every two hours not only at night but also during the day. This is because the feeding pattern of the previous 2–3 weeks has affected the supply of breast milk. Because the baby is feeding so often it is inevitable that, more often than not, the baby is being fed to sleep. This can often lead to long-term sleeping problems for many babies.

After months of sleepless nights and exhausting days with the baby still nursing every two or three hours, many parents ask their pediatrician for help. Or they purchase one or several of the many baby books on how to get your baby to sleep through the night, only to learn they got it all wrong in the first place. The real reason their baby is unable to sleep well is that he has had the wrong associations with going to sleep, i.e. feeding, rocking, patting, etc.

How well your baby sleeps is very closely linked to how well he feeds and what he associates with falling asleep. To encourage healthy sleep habits in your baby, it is important that you structure his feeding and have an understanding of the sleep rhythms of young babies, so that you establish the right sleep associations from very early on.

An understanding of sleep rhythms will also help you adjust the routines to suit the individual needs of your baby and, at times, to suit the occasions when it has not been possible to follow the routines to the letter.

Sleep Rhythms

According to the American Academy of Family Physicians, a newborn baby will sleep approximately 16 hours a day in the first few weeks. This sleep is broken into a series of short and longer periods. In the early days, sleep is very much linked to the baby's need to feeding little and often. It can take well up to an hour to feed, burp and change the baby, after which time he falls quickly into a deep sleep. If the baby has eaten well he will often sleep through to the next feeding. Over a 24-hour period, therefore, with the baby feeding 6–8 times a day and each feeding lasting between 45 minutes and one hour, the baby ends up sleeping approximately 16 hours a day.

However, between the third and fourth week, the baby becomes more alert and will not fall straight into a deep sleep after feeding. This is often a time when things start to go wrong, and the wrong sleep associations are developed. The anxious parents, believing that the baby should fall asleep straight after eating, start to resort to feeding, rocking or giving the baby a pacifier to induce sleep. They do not realize that it is around this age that the different stages of sleep become more apparent.

Like adults, babies drift from light sleep into a dreamlike sleep known as REM sleep, then into a deep sleep. The cycle is much shorter than that of an adult, lasting approximately 45 minutes to one hour. While some babies only stir when they drift into light sleep, others will wake fully. If the baby is due a feeding, this does not create a problem. However, if it has been only one hour since the baby ate last and the baby does not learn to settle himself, a real problem can develop over the months ahead if the baby is constantly assisted back to sleep. Recent research has shown that all babies drift into light sleep and wake approximately the same number of times during the night. Only the poor sleepers are unable to drift back into deep sleep, because they are used to being helped to sleep.

If you want your baby to develop good sleeping habits from an early age, it is important to avoid the wrong sleep associations. My routines are structured so that your baby eats well, never becomes overtired and does not learn the wrong associations when going to sleep.

· · · · · · · · · · ·

The Bedtime Routine

Once your baby has regained his birth weight and is gaining weight steadily, you can look at establishing a regular bedtime of 6:30–7 p.m., and allow him to sleep past the 9 p.m. feeding, feeding him at around 10 p.m. instead, pushing forward to 10:30 p.m. It is also at this stage that he should manage to sleep slightly longer in the night. If he eats well and settles at around 11–11:30 p.m., he will hopefully manage to sleep to between 2–3 a.m. If he feeds well then and settles back within an hour, he should manage to sleep until around 6–7 a.m., provided that he has been awakened enough for a full portion at the late feeding. During the early days, how soon babies wake after midnight is very much dependent upon how awake they were at the late feeding and how much they take then. It is worthwhile spending some time at this feeding to ensure that the baby does start to sleep a longer stretch in the night.

· · · · ·

Establishing a good bedtime routine and getting your baby to sleep well between 7–10 p.m. is a major factor in how quickly he will sleep through the night. A baby who eats well at 6 p.m. and settles to sleep well between 7 p.m. and 10 p.m. will wake refreshed and ready for a full feeding. However, there are other factors in establishing a regular bedtime routine. The main ones are that you have structured his eating and sleeping pattern during the day, so that he is hungry enough for a full feeding at 5–6:15 p.m.; and that he has been awake enough during the day, so he is ready to sleep at 7 p.m.

I get many calls and e-mails from parents who are struggling to settle their babies in the evening. When a pattern of feeding on and off occurs during the evening, in most cases it results in the baby not being hungry enough at the late feeding. The baby then ends up waking hungry around 1 a.m. and usually again at 4–5 a.m.

Establishing a bedtime routine will only be possible if your baby is well fed and ready to sleep by 6:30–7 p.m. For example, if you allow your baby to sleep for lengthy periods in the late afternoon, he is unlikely to settle well at 7 p.m.

The key to encouraging your baby to sleep well at night depends upon what happens during the day. Once he is gaining weight steadily, it means he is growing well. As he grows, the amount that he can take at each feeding should increase, and he should gradually be able to go longer between some feedings. Ideally, this longer spell should be between 7 p.m. and 10 p.m., and after the late and the middle-of-the-night feedings.

This will not necessarily happen automatically, which takes us back to what you may find the hardest part of the routines: waking your baby for daytime feedings at the recommended times for his age. But it is simply common sense that if your baby has fed regularly during the day, he should, as he grows, need to eat less during the night as the amount that he takes during the day increases.

Try, whenever possible, to start the day at 7 a.m. Stick to the times I advise in the routines and ensure that your baby takes a full feeding at those times and is awake for short periods after the daytime feedings. This will help you establish a bedtime routine in which your baby settles well at 7 p.m. Remember, if your baby eats and settles well by 7 p.m. and sleeps soundly until the late feeding, he will be much more likely to start to sleep longer in the night after that feeding, provided that he has been awake enough to eat until he is full.

As infants overtire easily, start the bedtime routine no later than 6 p.m. If your baby has not slept well at nap times you may need to start earlier. Keep things very calm and quiet throughout the bath, and after the bath avoid lots of eye contact and talking, so that he does not become overstimulated. Try always to do the last part of the feeding in a quiet, dimly lit room, so that you can quickly settle your baby in his bed before he falls into a deep sleep.

It will be difficult, but all the parents I have spoken to say that it was worth putting in the hard work in those early days, as their babies started to sleep longer and longer in the night, until they eventually made it through to that magical time of 7 a.m.

Early-morning Waking

I have always believed that whether a child becomes an early-morning waker is very much determined by what happens during the first year. In order to avoid this problem, it is crucial that the baby sleeps at night in a very dark room and that the parent treats any feedings before 7 a.m. as nighttime feedings.

They should be done with the minimum of fuss, with no talking or eye contact, and the baby should be settled back to sleep until 7 a.m. If your baby has woken between 6 a.m. and 6:30 a.m., then feed him and leave him until 7:30 a.m.

This approach has worked for the hundreds of babies I have helped care for, none of whom ever got up before 7 a.m., once they were sleeping through the night. Certainly some of these babies would wake around 5–6 a.m., perhaps chatter or sing for a short spell, then return to sleep.

Since the publication of the first edition of this book I have spoken to many parents who have experienced problems with early-morning waking. One thing that nearly all these parents had in common is that they did not follow my advice of allowing their babies to wake naturally. Most admitted to picking their babies up the minute they started to wake from daytime naps. Over time, it is not surprising that these babies came to expect the same thing to happen when they woke early in the morning.

Somewhere between 8 and 12 weeks, the majority of babies do not wake from naps immediately looking for food. This is a good time to encourage them to lie in their crib for a short time after waking. I am convinced that by doing this along with the following guidelines, there will be less chance of your baby becoming an early-morning riser:

* Research shows that the chemicals in the brain work differently in the dark, preparing it for sleep. From 6 months, when your baby can be put to sleep in his nursery, check that there are no chinks of light at the top or sides of the curtains or around the door. Even the smallest amount of light can be enough to wake the baby fully when he comes into a light sleep. It would be

worth investing in blackout lining for the nursery as well as for your bedroom where he will sleep at night for the first six months.

✳ Until babies reach six months, the "Moro reflex" can be quite strong and is very obvious in the early days. The baby flings his arms and legs back in jerky movements, usually if he gets shocked, is startled by a sudden loud noise or is put down too roughly or too quickly. The Moro reflex is also referred to as the "startle reflex."

As the weeks go by and the baby becomes more relaxed, the Moro reflex is less frequent. But it can take up to 7 or 8 months before it disappears altogether. I have observed many babies coming into their light sleep in the middle of the night and thrashing their legs up and down hysterically because they have kicked off their covers.

For this reason I believe it is very important that until the Moro reflex has totally disappeared, a baby is tucked in very securely by his bedcovers. The sheet and blankets should be placed lengthways across the width of the crib and then two rolled hand towels pushed down between the slats and the mattress to ensure that the bedding stays in place.

✳ Do not try to push your baby through the night by cutting down on his middle-of-the-night feeding. Continue to give him as much as he wants in the middle of the night to ensure that he sleeps soundly until 7 a.m. It is only when he has been sleeping regularly to 7 a.m. for a period of time and wakes refusing to feed well at 7 a.m., that you should consider cutting down the amount he is taking in the middle of the night.

✳ If your baby is feeding at 5–6 a.m., treat it as a night feeding. It should be done as quickly as possible in a dimly lit room without any eye contact or talking. Only change his diaper if necessary.

✳ Do not drop the late feeding until your baby is established on solid food. If he goes through a growth spurt before he starts his solids, he can be offered extra milk at this feeding. This reduces the chances of him waking early due to hunger.

. . . .

Your Questions Answered

Q How many hours of sleep a day does my newborn baby need?

A Depending upon weight and whether the baby was premature, most babies need 16–20 hours a day, broken into a series of short and long periods.

✳ Smaller babies and premature babies tend to need more sleep and will be more likely to doze on and off between feedings.

✳ Larger babies are capable of staying awake for an hour or so and sleeping for at least one longer spell of 4–5 hours during a 24-hour period.

✳ By the age of one month, most babies who are feeding well and gaining weight steadily are capable of sleeping for one longer stretch of 5–6 hours between feedings.

Q How do I make sure that the longer stretch of sleeping is always in the night and not during the day?

. . . . . .

A   Follow my routines and always start your day no later than 7 a.m., so that you have enough time to fit in all the feedings before 11 p.m.

* Keep your baby awake for at least 6–8 hours between 7 a.m. and 7 p.m.

* Always distinguish between sleep and awake time. During the first few weeks, ensure that the area where your baby is sleeping is kept as quiet as possible.

* Do not overstimulate your baby with lots of talking or eye contact during the feedings between 7 p.m. and 7 a.m.

Q   **I am trying to stick to your routines, but my four-week-old baby can only stay awake for an hour at the most after feedings. Should I be trying to make him stay awake longer?**

A   If your baby is eating well and gaining weight steadily, sleeping well between feedings in the night and alert for some of his awake periods during the day, then he is just one of those babies who needs more sleep.

* If he is waking more than twice in the night or staying awake for more than an hour in the night despite eating well at the late feeding, try stimulating him a bit more during the day.

* While the late feeding should always be a quiet one, an infant less than three months needs to be awake for at least 45 minutes. A sleepy feeding at this time will most certainly result in a baby being more awake around 2–3 a.m.

✳ If you structure your baby's eating and sleep times between 7 a.m. and 11 p.m. by my routines, when your baby does cut back on his sleep, it will be at the right time.

Q The routine seems very restricting. If I go out with my four-week-old during waking time he goes straight to sleep in the stroller, which means he has slept too much.

A Whether your baby is in my routine or not, during the first couple of months life is restrictive due to the amount of time spent nursing.

✳ By two months, most babies are capable of going longer between feedings and are faster eaters. This makes going out easier.

✳ For the first two months, if you plan your activities to fit around his sleep time, by eight weeks he will be able to stay awake longer when you take him out in the car or stroller.

Q My four-week-old baby has suddenly started to wake at 9 p.m. If I nurse him then, he wakes twice in the night, at 1 a.m. and 5 a.m. I have tried encouraging him to hold out until 10:30 p.m., but then he is so tired he doesn't eat properly, which means he still wakes earlier.

A Around one month, the light and deep sleep becomes much more defined. I find that a lot of babies come into a very light sleep around 9 p.m., so ensure that the area around where your baby is sleeping is kept as quiet as possible.

- Breast-fed babies may need a top-up of expressed milk after the 6 p.m. feeding.
- If you have to feed him at 9 p.m., settle him back to sleep with one breast or a couple of ounces, and then push the 10:30 p.m. feeding to 11:30 p.m. Hopefully, he will then take a full amount, which would get him through to 3:30 a.m.
- Alternatively, try giving a split feeding. Offer your baby a feeding at 9:30 p.m. and then keep him awake until you offer a further feeding at 10:30 p.m.

Q **I always have to wake my baby of 10 weeks for his late feeding, then he only takes 3–4 oz. and wakes again at 4 a.m. Could I just drop the last feeding and see if he goes through until 4 a.m. without that feeding?**

A I would not advise getting rid of the feeding yet, as he could wake at 1 a.m. and then 5 a.m., which, in effect, would be two night wakings. I have always found it best to get the baby sleeping through to 7 a.m. and taking solids before dropping the late feeding. This usually happens at about six months.

- Make sure he is tucked in properly; often a baby getting out of his blankets and thrashing around in his light sleep is enough to arouse him to a fully awake state. (See Chapter One, Preparation for the Birth, for advice on how to tuck your baby in properly.) If he is not getting out of his covers, I would wait 5–10 minutes before going to him, and then I would try settling him with some water. If he settles with the water he will make up for the lost feeding during the day and at his age the increased daily milk intake usually has the unintended consequence of him not needing to eat in the night. If he does not go back to sleep after the water, I would nurse him with a full feeding and try again in a couple of weeks.

* To encourage your baby to drink more at the late feeding and sleep longer in the night it may be worth introducing a split feeding. For this to work well you should start to wake your baby at around 9:45 p.m., so he is fully awake and eating by 10 p.m. Allow him to drink as much as he would want, then allow him time to play for a while on the floor on his play mat. At 11 p.m. you should then take him to the bedroom and change his diaper, then offer him a further feeding. If you are formula-feeding, I would advise that you make a fresh bottle for the second feed.

5

Establishing the Contented Little Baby Routines

· · · · · ·

The times for feeding and sleeping change 10 times during the first year of the CLB routines to ensure that the individual needs of every baby can be properly met. It is very important that you carefully read the advice and information in the feeding and sleeping chapters before you even attempt to start the routines. They will help you understand how best to use the routines so that your baby is happy, content, and eating and sleeping well.

After the birth follow the advice given for a newborn until he has regained his birth weight and shows signs of being able to go longer between feedings. Then you can move on to the first routine. Gradually, when your baby shows signs of going longer between feedings and staying awake longer, you can move on to the next routine. Do not worry if your baby is not managing the routine for his age; just stick to the routine that he is happy in and continue to watch for the signs that he is content and able to go longer between feedings and stay awake longer. Then move on to the next routine.

If you are starting the routines with an older baby who has established a pattern of demand-feeding and sleeping, look through the routines and find the one nearest to the pattern he is in now. Follow that routine for a short period and then, once he is eating and feeding happily at the times in that routine, you can move on to the next routine, gradually working your way through the different routines until he eventually reaches the one suitable for his age.

Feeding

Small babies spend a great deal of their waking time eating. To avoid excessive night feeding, it is important to structure and establish a good daytime pattern. As I have explained, in order to establish a good milk supply I believe that your baby needs to be fed little and often. The success of the CLB routines depends upon the baby being woken for feedings and not being left for long spells in between feedings. I recommend that in the very early days an every three-hours-feeding routine be established. This time is calculated from the beginning of one feeding to the beginning of the next. Of course, if a baby is demanding milk before the recommended time, I have always advised that he should be fed. But if this continues long after the milk has come in, then it is important to look for reasons why your baby is not lasting longer between feedings.

Only once a baby has regained his birth weight and continues to have a steady weight gain, do I recommend that the times between feedings should be extended and only if the baby shows signs of happily going longer between feedings. By structuring your baby's feedings from early on, things should never get to a stage at which he is having to cry to let you know he is hungry, as you will already be preempting his feeding needs.

From the very beginning, it is important to differentiate between feeding, sleeping and social times. If you talk too much or overstimulate him while feeding, he could lose interest after a couple of ounces, and then may not settle well into sleep. This could result in you feeding him to sleep, which in the long term can create sleep problems. Also avoid talking on the telephone for long periods while feeding.

It is important during the very early days that you concentrate on the positioning of your baby on the breast to ensure that he feeds well. Do seek help from a lactation consultant to make sure that you are getting the feeding position right. If you nurse him in a rocking chair, do not be tempted to rock him while feeding, as he will think it is sleep time, and if he is sleepy while feeding, he will not eat so well and will need to nurse again sooner. Sleepy babies are also often more prone to spitting up.

The aim of the CLB feeding routines is to ensure that when your baby is ready to increase the amount of milk he drinks, you structure his daytime feedings to correspond with his daytime sleep. This will mean that, as soon as your baby is physically and mentally capable, he will sleep his longest spell in the night and not during the day.

Sleeping

It is essential for your baby's mental and physical development that he gets enough sleep; without the right amount, he will become irritable, fretful and inconsolable. A baby who is constantly tired will not eat effectively and, therefore, not sleep properly. As I have already mentioned, one of the most important things that you should remember in the early days is that very young babies can only stay awake for **up to two hours** before becoming tired. If your baby stays awake for longer than two hours he could become so exhausted that he will need a much longer sleep at his next nap time. This will have a domino effect, altering the rest of his routine, resulting in poor evening and nighttime sleep. Therefore, it is essential that you structure the awake period properly, so that the feeding and sleeping plan works well. In the early days, some babies can only stay awake for an hour after eating; this is fairly normal for babies who need more sleep.

To determine whether your baby is a sleepy baby or not, consider his nighttime sleep pattern. If he can stay awake for only an hour at a time during the day but settles well in the evening and eats and settles quickly during the night, then he is a baby who needs more sleep. He will eventually manage to stay awake for longer amounts of time, provided you ensure that he is given the opportunity. You can do this by trying whenever possible to settle him in a quiet room for naps and having him in a bright, social and noisier environment during his waking time. Create the contrast between nap and social time to help him learn when it's time to sleep and when it's time to play.

However, if he can stay awake for only an hour at a time during the day but for several hours during the night, it is possible that he has his day and night confused, and it is worthwhile encouraging him to stay awake more during the day. Babies learn by association. It is very important that from day one he learns the right associations and to differentiate between eating, playing, cuddling and sleeping.

You will also find that there are some times of the day when your baby will stay awake for two hours quite happily and other times when he will be tired after an hour. This is perfectly normal in the early days, which is why I say that babies can stay awake for *up to* two hours—not that they *must* stay awake for two hours.

Along with the routines, the following guidelines will help your baby develop healthy sleeping habits:

* Keep him awake for a short spell after his day feedings.
* Do not let him sleep too long in the late afternoon.
* Do not feed him after 3:15 p.m., as it will throw off his next feeding.
* Follow the same routine every evening; do not allow visitors around the baby during wind-down time.
* Do not let him get overtired; allow at least one hour for the bath, feeding and winding-down time.
* Do not overstimulate him or play with him after his bath.
* Do not rock him to sleep in your arms; settle him in his crib before he goes into a deep sleep.
* If you use a pacifier to calm him down, remove it before you put him in his crib.
* If he falls asleep on the breast or bottle, arouse him slightly before settling him in his crib.

Playing

All babies love to be cuddled and talked and sung to. Research also shows that even very small babies like to look at simple books and interesting toys. For your baby to enjoy these things, it is important that you do them at the right time. The best time is usually approximately one hour after he is awake and has been fed. He should never be played with or overstimulated 20 minutes before his nap. Imagine how you would feel if you were just drifting off to sleep and someone came into the room and wanted to laugh and joke with you. I doubt you would be too happy about it, so respect that your baby needs the same quiet time before he goes off to sleep.

Pay particular attention to what toys your baby gets used to in his crib. I find it a great help to divide toys and books into wake-up and winding-down ones. Musical crib mobiles and colorful baby gyms, plus black-and-white cloth crib books are all excellent for keeping young babies interested for short spells, during social time, as are postcards and posters that show single objects or faces. Use these toys only during social times and two or three different, less stimulating toys for winding-down times.

Babies have very short concentration spans; constantly talking and handling a baby during the social time can often result in him becoming overstimulated. It's important to take the cue from your baby as to how much stimulation he can handle. Even from a very young age, babies should be encouraged to occupy themselves for short periods and have freedom to move. This is much more likely to happen if the baby is allowed to lie on his play mat or under his crib mobile, as he will be able to kick and move around more than when he is being held.

. . . .

Cuddling

Babies need lots of cuddling, but it should always be done when your baby needs it, not when *you* need it. A baby needs energy to grow, so it is important that you do not overhandle his small body and exhaust him. While all babies need to be nurtured, they are not toys. Differentiate the type of cuddle during his playtime from that of winding-down time. Winding-down cuddling should be about closeness of bodies. It is important that your baby is not cuddled to sleep while feeding. After one hour of being awake and fed he should be happy to spend a little time amusing himself; if you constantly cuddle him during playtime, he will be less likely to respond to the cuddles that would normally help settle him for his nap. When cuddling him during the winding-down time, do not talk and avoid eye contact, as it can overstimulate him and result in him becoming overtired and not settling. Instead, just enjoy that peaceful connection and closeness that you feel with him.

Structuring the Milk Feedings During the First Year

During the first few weeks, regardless of whether babies are breast- or formula-fed, very few can manage a strict every-four-hour-feeding pattern, and the aim of the CLB feeding routines is to ensure that the individual needs of all babies can be met. That is why I recommend that babies are fed every three hours in the early days, and only when they have regained their birth weight and are gaining weight steadily should they be left to go longer for feedings. By two weeks, if your baby has regained his birth weight and weighs more than 7 lbs., he should manage to last 3–4 hours between some feedings, provided he is drinking the full amount at the times stated in the routines. By structuring feedings in the early days, you can achieve several slots of every-three-hours feedings and some of a four-hour stretch. If you structure his feedings according to the routines, the four-hour stretch between feedings should always happen between

10 a.m. and 2 p.m. and 7 p.m. and 7 a.m. This would mean that a baby who ate at 6 p.m. should get to 10 p.m., and then eat again around 2–3 a.m., then again at 5/6–7 a.m.

The three-hour stretch between feedings is timed from the beginning of one feeding to the beginning of the next; a baby starting to feed at 7 a.m. would then need to start his next feeding at 10 a.m. However, if you feel your baby is genuinely hungry before his next feeding is due, as I have mentioned earlier, he must be fed—but it is also advisable to get to the root of the problem as to why he is not taking a full feeding at the times stated in the routines. If you are nursing, it may be that he needs longer on the second breast; if you are bottle-feeding, it may be that he needs an extra ounce at some feedings.

Between the second and fourth week, most babies who are gaining weight steadily are able to last slightly longer after one feeding—usually 4½–5 hours. If you structure your baby's feedings, this will automatically be at the right time, i.e., between 11 p.m. and 7 a.m.

If your baby has been demand-fed and you are attempting to put him into a routine, I advise that you look at the early routines and put him into a routine that seems nearest to his demand-fed pattern. For example, a nine-week-old baby may need to start on the 2–4 week schedule. When he is happy in that routine, you should be able to work your way through the next two sets of routines within 7–10 days. By the time he reaches 12 weeks, he should be happily eating at the times stated in the routine for his age. However, although it may take slightly longer for him to sleep through the night, the important thing is that he is only feeding once in the night and gradually increasing the length of time he sleeps from his last feeding, over a period of several weeks. Once the baby starts to sleep longer in the night, it is important to keep a close eye on how you structure feedings, as things can go wrong, particularly if you have been *too* strict. Remember the whole key to the CLB feeding routines is that they are flexible and that no baby should ever be forced to go longer before feeding than he is physically capable of.

The following extract is from the diary of a mother with a five-week-old baby going approximately four hours between feedings. It shows how quickly things can go wrong, when a strict routine of feeding every four hours is followed.

Tues	3 a.m.	7 a.m.	11 a.m.	3 p.m.	7 p.m.	11 p.m.
Wed	3 a.m.	7 a.m.	11 a.m.	3 p.m.	7 p.m.	11 p.m.
Thurs	4 a.m.	8 a.m.	12 p.m.	4 p.m.	8 p.m.	12 a.m.
Fri	5 a.m.	9 a.m.	1 p.m.	5 p.m.	9 p.m.	11 p.m.
Sat	2 a.m.	6 a.m.	10 a.m.	2 p.m.	6 p.m.	10 p.m.
Sun	2 a.m.	6 a.m.	10 a.m.	2 p.m.	6 p.m.	10 p.m.

Aware that her baby's eating pattern was going haywire, the mother tried to get it back on track on the Friday night by waking the baby up at 11 p.m. This did not work, as the baby had taken a full feeding at 9 p.m. and was not hungry. The results were so poor that the baby woke up at 2 a.m. needing a full feeding, which meant a total backtrack on night feeding. Even if the mother had managed to settle the baby at 9 p.m. with a smaller feeding, it is unlikely the baby would have eaten any better. The baby had only been asleep for one hour so it would have been very difficult to wake him up enough to nurse properly.

As I mentioned earlier, the easiest way to keep your baby on track is to wake him at 7 a.m. Once he is sleeping to 5 a.m. or 6 a.m., he should be offered a top-up feeding at 7 a.m. or 7:30 a.m. This method will not only keep the rest of your feedings on track, but also ensure that your baby's sleeping is kept on track and that he is ready to go to bed at 7 p.m.

The following advice will also ensure that your baby sleeps through the night as soon as he is physically able, and prepare him for the introduction of solids and the eventual reduction of milk feedings.

. . . .

Understanding the Routines for Feeding

The 6–7 A.M. Feeding

* Depending upon what time he ate during the night, your baby will probably wake between 6 a.m. and 7 a.m., but he should always be woken at 7 a.m. regardless. Remember that one of the main keys to getting your baby to sleep through the night is to ensure that once he is physically capable of taking bigger amounts, he gets his daily requirements between 7 a.m. and 11 p.m.

* Regardless of whether he is breast- or bottle-fed, the only way to keep a baby in a good routine is to begin the day at 7 a.m. Once he is sleeping through the night, he should be at his hungriest at this feeding.

* During growth spurts, breast-fed babies should be given longer on the breast to ensure that their increased needs are met. If you have been expressing, you can increase this by 1 oz. If you have not been expressing, you can still follow the feeding times from the routine for your baby's age; just top him up with a short breast-feed before his daytime naps. If you do this for a week or so, this should help increase your milk supply. A sign that this has happened is that your baby will sleep well during his naps and not be so interested in the next feeding.

. . . . . .

BY SEVEN MONTHS

* If your baby is eating a full breakfast of cereal, fruit and perhaps small pieces of toast, you should aim to cut back the amount offered to him from the breast or bottle. Divide the milk between the drink and the cereal. Always encourage him to take at least 5–6 oz. before he is given his solids.

* If you are still nursing, gradually reduce the time he is on the first breast, then give him his solids and, finally, a further short feeding from the second breast. Keep a very close watch that you do not allow him to increase his solids so much that he cuts back too much on his breast-feeding.

* Your baby still needs a minimum of 20 oz. a day, inclusive of milk used in cooking or on cereal, divided between 3 or 4 milk feedings.

BY TEN MONTHS

* If your baby is formula-fed, encourage him to drink all his milk from a cup. Ensure that you still offer milk at the start of the meal. Once he has taken 5–6 oz. of his milk, offer him some cereal. Then offer him the remainder of his milk again.

* It is important that he has at least 6–8 oz. of milk divided between the cup and the breakfast cereal.

* If you are still nursing, offer him first the breast then the solids, then offer him the breast again.

* Your baby needs a minimum of 18 oz. a day, inclusive of milk used in cooking or on cereal, divided between 2 or 3 milk feedings.

The 10–11 A.M. Feeding

✳ During the first few weeks, the majority of babies who have eaten between 6 a.m. and 7 a.m. will wake looking for a feeding around 10 a.m. Even if your baby does not do this, it is important that you wake him. Remember that the aim is to ensure that your baby feeds regularly during the day so that he only needs to wake once for a feeding between 11 p.m. and 6–7 a.m.

✳ In the early days, many babies would happily sleep 4–5 hours between feedings during the day. Regardless of whether a baby is breast-fed or bottle-fed, within a very short period, this usually leads to several nighttime feedings as the baby attempts to get all his daily nutritional needs. It also puts him at possible risk of dehydration.

✳ Too few feedings during the day in the early weeks also does little to help establish a good milk supply for a breast-feeding mother, and nursing several times a night soon exhausts the mother so much that her milk supply is reduced even further.

✳ Around six weeks, your baby may show signs of being happy to go longer from the 7 a.m. feeding, and the 10 a.m. feeding can gradually be pushed to 10:30 a.m. However, a baby who is eating at 5 a.m. or 6 a.m. and being topped up at 7:30 a.m. would probably still need to eat at 10 a.m., as would the baby who has too little to eat at 7 a.m.

✳ Once he is sleeping through the night, or taking only a small feeding in the night, he should have the biggest feeding of the day at 6:45–7 a.m. If he eats well, he should be happy to last until 11 a.m. before needing to eat again. However, if you feed him before he really needs it, he may not eat well and, as a result, may sleep poorly at the lunchtime nap. This will have a domino effect so that each subsequent feeding and nap has to be given earlier, and may result in the baby waking at 6 a.m. or earlier the following morning.

＊ This feeding would be the next one to be increased during growth spurts.

BY 6–7 MONTHS

＊ When your baby is eating breakfast, you can start to make this feeding later, eventually settling somewhere between 11:30 a.m. and noon. This will be the pattern for three meals a day at the end of six months, at which stage the milk feeding will be replaced with a drink of well-diluted juice or water from a cup.

＊ It is important that you introduce the tier system of feeding so that he gradually cuts back on the amount of milk he drinks and increases his intake of solids.

＊ Some babies simply refuse to cut back on their milk intake at this feeding. If you find that your baby is one, please refer to Chapter Sixteen, Problem Solving in the First Year, for suggestions.

BY SEVEN MONTHS

＊ Once your baby is on a fully balanced diet of solids, which includes protein with lunch, it is important that this feeding be replaced with a drink of water or well-diluted juice. Formula given with a protein meal can reduce the iron absorption by up to 50 percent.

＊ Give the baby most of his solids before his drink so he doesn't fill up with liquid first.

THE 2:30 P.M. FEEDING

* During the first few months, make this feeding smaller so that your baby eats really well at the 5–6:15 p.m. feeding, the exception being that if your baby doesn't sleep well at lunchtime, he will need to eat earlier with a top-up at 2:30 p.m. If, for some reason, the baby eats poorly at the 10 a.m. feeding or was fed earlier, increase this feeding accordingly so that he maintains his daily milk quota.

* If your baby is very hungry and regularly drains the bottle at this feeding, then you can give him the full amount, provided he does not take less at the next feeding.

* For breast-fed babies, allow longer on the breast if he is not managing to get happily to the next feeding.

BY EIGHT MONTHS

* When your baby is having three full solid meals a day and his lunchtime milk feeding has been replaced with water or well-diluted juice, you will probably need to increase this feeding so that he is getting his daily milk quota in three milk feedings.

* However, if he cuts back on the last milk feeding of the day, it would be advisable to keep this milk feeding smaller and make the daily quota by using milk in cereals and cooking.

* Your baby still needs a minimum of 18–20 oz. a day, inclusive of milk used in cooking and on cereal.

BY 9–12 MONTHS

* Bottle-fed babies should be given their milk from a cup at this stage, which should automatically result in a decrease in the amount they drink.

✳ If this is not the case and your baby starts to lose interest in his morning or evening feeding, you could cut back on this feeding. If he is getting 18–20 oz. of milk a day (inclusive of milk used in cooking and on cereal), plus a well-balanced diet of solids, you could cut this feeding altogether.

✳ By one-year-old, your baby needs a minimum of 12 oz. a day, inclusive of milk used in cooking and cereal.

The 6–7 P.M. Feeding

✳ It is important that your baby always has a good feeding at this time if you want him to settle down well between 7 p.m. and 10 p.m.

✳ He should not be fed milk after 3:15 p.m., as it could put him off taking a good feeding later in the evening.

✳ In the first few weeks, this feeding is split between 5 p.m. and 6:15 p.m. so that the baby does not get too frantic during his bath. Once your baby has slept through the night for two weeks, the 5 p.m. feeding can be dropped. I would not recommend dropping the split feeding until this happens, as a larger feeding at 6:15 p.m. could result in your baby taking even less at the last feeding, resulting in an earlier waking time. With many of the babies that I cared for, I continued to give them a split feeding until solids were introduced to ensure that they were getting enough milk during the day. Once you eliminate the 5 p.m. feeding and your baby is taking a full feeding after the bath, he could cut down dramatically on his last feeding of the day, which could result in an early waking.

✳ Breast-fed babies not settling at 7 p.m. should be offered a top-up of expressed milk. Your milk supply may well be low at this time of the day.

BY 4–5 MONTHS

✳ If your baby has started solids early, he should be given most of his milk before his solids, as milk is still the most important form of nutrition at this age.

✳ Most babies will be taking a full breast or bottle-feeding at this age.

✳ If he is weaned and very tired when he eats, and you are struggling to get him to drink all of his milk plus any solids you have been advised to introduce, adjust the feeding times. Try giving two-thirds of each milk feeding at around 5:30 p.m. followed by his solids, then delay his bath until around 6:25 p.m. After the bath he can then be offered the remainder of his milk feeding. If formula feeding, it is advisable to make two separate bottles to ensure that the milk is fresh.

✳ A breast-fed baby who has reached five months, is being weaned and is now starting to wake before 10:30 p.m. may not be getting enough milk at this time. Try giving a full breast-feed at 5:30 p.m. followed by the solids, with a bath at 6:15 p.m., followed by a top-up of expressed milk or formula after the bath. A baby who is not weaned would more than likely need to continue to have a split-milk feeding at 5–6:15 p.m. until solids are introduced.

BY 6–7 MONTHS

✳ Most babies will now be having supper at 5 p.m. followed by a full breast-feed or a full formula-feed. Once solids are established and the late feeding is dropped, you may find that if you are breast-feeding, your baby starts to wake earlier. I suggest that if this happens you offer a top-up of expressed milk to ensure that he settles well at 7 p.m. and sleeps until morning.

BY 10–12 MONTHS

✻ Bottle-fed babies should be taking all of their milk from a cup at one year. Babies who continue to feed from a bottle after this age are more prone to feeding problems, as they continue to take large amounts, which takes the edge off their appetite for solids.

✻ Start encouraging your baby to take some of his milk from a cup at 10 months, so that by one year he is happy to take all of his last feeding from a cup.

The Late Feeding

✻ I strongly advise that parents of breast-fed babies should introduce bottles of either expressed milk or formula at this feeding and do it no later than the second week. This will help the primary caregiver share the feeding responsibilities with a partner.

✻ This also helps to avoid the common problem of a baby refusing to take a bottle at a later stage.

✻ A totally breast-fed baby less than three months who continues to wake between 2–3 a.m. and shows no sign of going for a longer stretch in the night may not be getting enough to eat at this time, as the breast-milk supply is often at its lowest at this time of day.

✻ If you choose to top-up with expressed milk or formula rather than completely replacing the feeding with a full bottle-feeding, it is essential to make sure your baby has completely emptied the breast before he is offered the top-up feed.

* It is easier to tell whether formula-fed babies are getting enough to eat at this feeding. If you always increase the day feedings during your baby's growth spurts, he will probably never require more than 6 oz. at this feeding. However, babies who weighed more than 10 lbs. at birth may reach a stage at which they need more than this—at least until they are well established on solids.

* Refer to Chapter Three, Milk Feeding in the First Year, for calculating how much formula your baby needs each day, and for how to structure the feedings.

BY 3–4 MONTHS

* If your baby has slept through the night until 7 a.m. for at least two weeks, then you can bring this feeding forward by 10 minutes every three nights, until your baby is sleeping from 10 p.m. to 6:45–7 a.m.

* If your baby is totally breast-fed and is still waking early in the night, despite being topped up with expressed milk at the late feeding, it may be worthwhile talking to your doctor about replacing the late breast-feeding with a formula-feeding. Most formula-fed babies will be taking 7–8 oz. a feeding 4–5 times a day.

* If a formula-fed baby is not sleeping through the night at this age, it may be because he needs a little extra at this feeding, and even if it means he cuts back on what he eats in the morning, it may be worth offering him an extra ounce or two.

* Some babies simply refuse this feeding at 3–4 months. If your baby is eating well from the breast four times a day and your doctor is happy with his weight gain, you can just

drop this feeding. However, if you find that he starts to wake earlier again and will not settle back to sleep within 10 minutes or so, assume it might be hunger and feed him. You may then have to consider reintroducing the late feeding until he is weaned and established on solids.

✳ If your baby is waking twice in the night (i.e., 2 a.m. and 5 a.m.) or is not sleeping past 5 a.m., you can try waking the baby at 9:45 p.m. for this feeding. Ensure he is wide awake either by changing his diaper or by letting him play for a few minutes on his mat. Turn on all the lights. He should be ready to eat by 10 p.m. Feed him, then keep him up until 11 p.m. by changing him or playing (whichever you didn't do at 9:45 p.m.). Top him up just before he goes down at 11 p.m. By ensuring he is awake for longer at this feeding and splitting it, he should wake only once in the night. Once this is established and he is going for a longer spell at night, you can slowly move the whole of this feeding back to 10 or 10:15 p.m.

BY 4–7 MONTHS

✳ The majority of babies at this age should be capable of sleeping through the night from their last feeding, provided they are having their daily intake of milk between 7 a.m. and 11 p.m.

✳ A baby who is being exclusively breast-fed may only manage to get through to around 5 a.m. until he is weaned.

✳ Once your baby has been weaned and is established on three solid meals a day, this last feeding should gradually reduce automatically. This will depend upon how much solid food your baby is taking once he reaches 6–7 months. If you have been advised to wean your baby earlier than six months, you should find that you could drop this feeding fairly quickly once he reaches this age. A baby who did not start solids until the recommended age of six months may still need this feeding until he reaches seven months. By this time, provided the baby is taking enough milk and solids during the day, you should be able to gradually reduce the amount he takes and then eliminate it altogether.

THE 2–3 A.M. FEEDING

✳ Newborn babies need to feed little and often during the first week, so when they wake it is best to assume that they are hungry and feed them.

✳ A newborn baby should never be allowed to go longer than three hours between feedings during the day and four hours between feedings in the night. This time is measured from the beginning of one feeding to the beginning of the next.

✳ Once your baby has regained his birth weight, he should start to settle into the two- to four-week routine. Provided he eats well between 10 p.m. and 11 p.m., he should manage to sleep closer to 2 a.m.

BY 4–6 WEEKS

✳ Most babies gaining the right amount of weight each week are capable of lasting a longer stretch between feedings during the night, as long as

  * The baby is taking his daily allowance of milk in the five feedings between 7 a.m. and 11 p.m.
  * The baby is not sleeping more than 4½ hours between 7 a.m. and 7 p.m.

BY 6–8 WEEKS

✶ If your baby is gaining the right amount of weight each week but is still waking between 2 a.m. and 3 a.m., despite eating a good amount at the late feeding, settle him with some cool, boiled water. If he refuses to settle, you will have to feed him.

✶ If the baby does settle, he will probably wake again around 5 a.m., at which time you can give him a full feeding, followed by a top-up at 7–7:30 a.m. This will help keep him on track with his feeding and sleeping pattern for the rest of the day.

✶ Within a week, babies usually sleep until close to 5 a.m., gradually increasing their sleep time until 7 a.m. During this stage, when your baby is taking a top-up at 7–7:30 a.m. instead of a full feeding, he may not manage to get through to 10:45–11 a.m. for his next feeding. You may need to give him half the amount at 10 a.m. followed by the remainder at 10:45–11 a.m., followed by a top-up just before he goes down for his lunchtime nap, to ensure that he does not wake early from the nap.

BY 3–4 MONTHS

✶ Both breast fed and bottle fed babies should be able to go for one long spell during the night by this age, provided they are getting their daily intake of milk between 6/7 a.m. and 10/11 p.m.

✶ Your baby should be sleeping no more than three hours between 7 a.m. and 7 p.m.

✶ If your baby insists on waking before 4/5 a.m. in the night, refuses cool boiled water and will not settle without eating, keep a very detailed diary listing exact times and amounts of feeding and times of daytime naps. A baby who cuts back on his 7 a.m. feeding could be waking out of habit rather than hunger.

＊ Some breast-fed babies may still genuinely need to nurse in the night if they are not getting enough at their late feeding. If you are not already doing so, it is worth considering a top-up feeding of expressed milk or formula, or a replacement formula feeding at the late feeding.

＊ Whether you are breast-feeding or bottle-feeding, if your baby's weight gain is good, you are convinced he is waking from habit and he refuses cool boiled water, try leaving him for 15–20 minutes before going to him. Some babies will grumble on and off and then settle themselves back to sleep.

＊ A baby of this age may still be waking in the night because he is getting out of his covers. Try tucking him in using two rolled-up towels wedged between the mattress and the slats of the crib to keep the sheet firm.

BY 4–5 MONTHS

If your baby reaches five months and is still waking in the night, you probably need to persevere with his routine, paying increased attention to the timings of the feedings and the amount of daytime sleep he is getting. If you feel that he is showing signs that he is ready to be weaned, consult your pediatrician for advice as to whether he should begin earlier than the recommended six months.

MILK FEEDING CHART FOR THE FIRST YEAR

AGE	TIMES
2–4 weeks	2–3 a.m. 6–7 a.m. 10–10:30 a.m. 2–2:30 a.m. 5 p.m. 6–6:30 p.m. 10–11 p.m.
4–6 weeks	3–4 a.m. 6–7 a.m. 10:30–11 a.m. 2–2:30 p.m. 5 p.m. 6–6:30 p.m. 10–11 p.m.
6–8 weeks	4–5 a.m. 7:30 a.m. 10:45–11 a.m. 2–2:30 p.m. 6–6:30 p.m. 10–11 p.m.
8–10 weeks	5–6 a.m. 7:30 a.m. 11 a.m. 2–2:30 p.m. 6–6:30 p.m. 10–11 p.m.
10–12 weeks	7 a.m. 11 a.m. 2–2:30 p.m. 6–6:30 p.m. 10–11 p.m.
3–4 months	7 a.m. 11 a.m. 2–2:30 p.m. 6–6:30 p.m. 10–10:30 p.m.
4–5 months	7 a.m. 11 a.m. 2–2:30 p.m. 6–6:30 p.m. 10 p.m.
5–6 months	7 a.m. 11:30 a.m. 2–2:30 p.m. 6–6:30 p.m.
6–7 months	7 a.m. 2–2:30 p.m. 6–6:30 p.m.
7–8 months	7 a.m. 2–2:30 p.m. 6–6:30 p.m.
8–9 months	7 a.m. 2–2:30 p.m. 6–6:30 p.m.
9–10 months	7 a.m. 5 p.m. 6:30–7 p.m.
10–12 months	7 a.m. 5 p.m. 6:30–7 p.m.

• • • • • • • • • • •

Structuring Daytime Sleep During the First Year

The whole aim of the CLB routines is to ensure that the timings of feedings fit in with your baby's daily sleep requirements. A baby who does not eat well during the day will not sleep well during the day; and to ensure good nighttime sleep for your baby it is essential that you structure his daytime sleep. Too much sleep can result in nighttime wakings. Too little can result in an overtired, irritable baby who has difficulty settling himself to sleep and who falls asleep only when he is totally exhausted.

When following the routines it is important to remember that they are guidelines to help you decide just how long your baby can stay awake before he needs to nap. In the routines, I stress that most babies in the early days can stay awake happily for **up**

• • • • • •

to two hours before needing a nap. I do not say that they *must* stay awake for the full two hours, only that it is important, if overtiredness is to be avoided, that they do not stay awake longer than two hours. So if, during the early days, you find that your baby is only staying awake for 1–1½ hours at a time, you do not need to worry as he is obviously a baby that needs more sleep, and as he grows, he will start to stay awake longer.

Of course, if you have a baby who is staying awake only an hour at a time during the day and partying for several hours in the night, this is a different matter, and you may have to try harder to encourage him to stay awake longer during the day, to avoid excessive nighttime waking.

The Importance of Nap Times

Infant sleep expert Marc Weissbluth, M.D., has carried out extensive research into the nap patterns of more than 200 children. He says that napping is one of the healthy habits that sets the stage for good overall sleep and explains that a nap offers the baby a break from stimuli and allows him to recharge for further activity. Charles Schaefer, Ph.D., Professor of Psychology at Fairleigh Dickinson University in Teaneck, New Jersey, supports this and says: "Naps structure the day, shape both the baby's and the mother's moods, and offer the only opportunity for Mom to relax or accomplish a few tasks."

Several leading experts on child care are in agreement that naps are essential to a baby's brain development. John Herman, Ph.D., infant sleep expert and Associate Professor of Psychology and Psychiatry at the University of Texas, says: "If activities are being scheduled to the detriment of sleep, it's a mistake. Parents should come after sleeping and eating." I couldn't agree more.

By 3–4 months, most babies are capable of sleeping 12 hours at night (with a sleepy feeding at 10 p.m.), provided their daytime sleep is no more than 3–3½ hours, divided between two or three naps a day. If you want your baby to sleep from 7–7:30 p.m. to 7–7:30 a.m., it is very important you structure these naps so that he has his longest nap at midday, with two shorter ones in the morning and late afternoon. While it may be more convenient to let your baby have a longer nap in the morning followed by a shorter nap in the afternoon, this can lead to problems as he gets older.

Once he reduces his daytime sleep naturally, he is most likely to cut back on his late-afternoon nap. His longest nap of the day would then be in the morning. By late afternoon, he will be exhausted and need to go to bed by 6:30 p.m. This could result in him waking at 6 a.m. If you manage to get him to have a nap in the late afternoon, you could then be faced with the problem of him not settling well at 7–7:30 p.m.

· · · · · · · · · · · ·

Understanding the Sleeping Routine

Morning Nap

Most babies are ready for a nap approximately two hours from the time they wake in the morning. This should always be a short nap, around 45–60 minutes. When he is between six and nine months, this nap can be shortened to 30 minutes and be closer to 10 a.m. Around 9–12 months, most babies will reduce the time of this nap or cut it out altogether. For some, this can happen as early as eight months, for others, as late as 18 months. You will know your baby is ready to drop this nap when he starts taking a long time to settle and ends up sleeping only 10–15 minutes of his 30–45 minute nap. Other telling signs that this nap may need to be cut down or perhaps dropped is when a baby is waking during his lunchtime nap, in the night or early morning, when he had previously slept well. If a baby is resisting sleep at his morning nap and for a couple of weeks manages to get through to his lunchtime nap happily, cut the morning nap out altogether. It is very important that you always start to wake him after the 30–45 minute period, even if he has only slept for 10 minutes. If you allow him to sleep past this time, you will not know whether he is ready to drop the nap. It could also cause him to sleep too little at his lunchtime nap and result in the problems discussed earlier.

SIX WEEKS ONWARD

Until a proper sleep pattern has been established, ensure that this nap takes place in a quiet room if possible. Once a proper daytime routine has been established, this nap could at times be taken in the stroller or car seat if you have to go out, but do remember to wake him after the 45 minutes.

If he is awake at 7 a.m., he may still need a 30-minute nap at 9:30 a.m. If you find that he is only sleeping 10–15 minutes and is getting through happily to his lunchtime nap, you could cut this nap out altogether. If he sleeps to 8 a.m., he should be able to get through to his lunchtime nap without the morning nap.

Lunchtime Nap

This should always be the longest sleep of the day. By establishing a good lunchtime nap, you will ensure that your baby is not too tired to enjoy afternoon activities and that bedtime is relaxed and happy. Recent research shows that a nap between noon and 2 p.m. is deeper and more refreshing than a later nap because it coincides with the baby's natural dip in alertness. As

I explained earlier, allowing a longer nap in the morning, followed by a shorter one at this time, will, in turn, affect the rest of his sleep, which can result in an early-morning awakening.

Most babies will need to sleep 2–2½ hours a day until they are 18–24 months old, when that time will gradually reduce to 1–1½ hours. By three years of age, they may not need a sleep after lunch, but they should always be encouraged to have some quiet time in their room. Otherwise, they are likely to get very hyperactive by late afternoon, which can affect the night sleep.

SIX WEEKS ONWARD

If your baby is sleeping the full 45 minutes in the morning, he should be woken after two hours. If, for some reason, his morning nap was much shorter, then you could allow him 2½ hours. If your baby develops a problem with his nighttime sleep, do not make the mistake of letting him sleep longer during the day.

In the early days, a lunchtime nap may sometimes go wrong, and your baby will refuse to go back to sleep. Obviously, he cannot make it through from 1 p.m. to 4 p.m. happily. I find the best way to deal with this is to allow 30 minutes after the 2:30 p.m. feeding, then a further 30 minutes at 4:30 p.m. This should stop him becoming overtired and irritable and get things back on track so that he goes to sleep well at 7 p.m. See Chapter Sixteen, Problem Solving in the First Year, for more in-depth help with this.

SIX MONTHS ONWARD

If your baby is on three meals a day, you should be aiming to move the morning nap from 9 a.m. to 9:30 a.m., and you will most likely need to adjust the lunchtime nap to 12:30–2:30

p.m. If he is sleeping less than two hours at lunchtime, check that his morning nap between 7 a.m. and noon is no more than 30 minutes.

TWELVE MONTHS ONWARD

If your baby has difficulty in settling for the nap or is waking after 1–1½ hours, you might have to cut the morning nap back or get rid of it altogether. Do not let him sleep after 2:30 p.m. if you want him to go to sleep at 7 p.m.

Late-afternoon Nap

This is the shortest nap of the three, and the one the baby should drop first. It is essential that your baby learn to sleep in places other than his bed as it also allows you the freedom to get out and about.

It is important that the late-afternoon nap is as close to 5 p.m. as possible in order to ensure that your baby is refreshed for his bath and bedtime routine. This will also have the domino effect of him settling well at 7 p.m. (as he will not be over-tired) and make it easier for you to wake him fully and take a good feeding at the late feeding. In the early days, if he is very sleepy after the 2 p.m. feeding, allow him a short catnap of about 20 minutes and then encourage him to have another short nap in his bassinet, stroller or car seat at 4:40–5 p.m.

THREE MONTHS ONWARD

If you want your baby to go to sleep at 7 p.m., he should never sleep more than 45 minutes at this nap, and he should always be awake by 5 p.m., regardless of how long or short his sleep was. Most babies who are sleeping well at the other two naps will gradually cut back on this sleep until they cut it out altogether. If, for some reason, his lunchtime nap was cut short, you would need to allow him a short sleep now but ensure that his daily total does not exceed the amount needed for his age.

. . . .

Adjusting the Routines

Birth to Six Months

I have tried many different routines over the years and, without exception, I have found the 7 a.m. to 7 p.m. routine to be the one in which tiny babies and young infants are happiest. It fits in with their natural sleep rhythms and their need to feed little and often. I urge parents to stick to the original routine whenever possible. Once your baby reaches the age of six months, is on four or five feedings a day and needs less sleep, it is possible to change the routine without affecting your baby's natural needs for the right amount of sleep and number of feedings.

Up to the age of six months, the following points should be noted when planning a routine:

✳ In the very early weeks, to avoid more than one waking in the night, you must fit in at least five feedings before midnight. This can only be done if your baby starts his day at 6–7 a.m.

✳ An 8 a.m. to 8 p.m. routine in the first few weeks would mean your baby would end up feeding twice between midnight and 7 a.m.

. . . . . .

Six Months Onward

From six months, when your baby has started solids and you have dropped the late feeding, it is easier to adjust the routine. If your baby has been sleeping regularly to 7 a.m., it could be possible to change to a 7:30 a.m. or 8 a.m. start and push the rest of the routine forward. Your baby would obviously need to go to sleep later in the evenings. If you want your baby to sleep later but still go to bed at 7 p.m., try the following:

* Cut back on the morning nap, so that your baby is ready to go to bed at 12–12:30 p.m.
* Allow a nap of no longer than two hours at lunchtime and no late-afternoon nap.

Out and About

In the first few weeks, most young babies will go to sleep the minute they are in the car or the stroller. If possible, organize trips away from home during the sleep times so that the routine is not too disrupted. Once the routine is established and your baby is closer to eight weeks old, you will find that you are able to go out more often without him falling asleep the whole time.

If you are planning a daylong excursion, depending upon the length of the planned event or appointment, you can usually work it into the routine by traveling between 9 a.m. and 10 a.m., or 1 p.m. and 2 p.m. By the time you arrive at the destination, the baby will be due for a feeding and can be kept awake. Likewise, by making the return journey between 4 p.m. and 5 p.m. or after 7 p.m., you should manage to keep things on track.

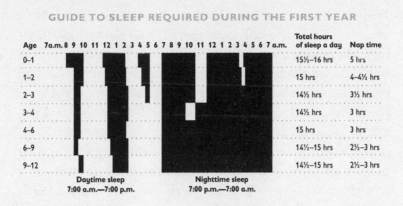

GUIDE TO SLEEP REQUIRED DURING THE FIRST YEAR

Age	7a.m.	8	9	10	11	12	1	2	3	4	5	6	7	8	9	10	11	12	1	2	3	4	5	6	7 a.m.	Total hours of sleep a day	Nap time
0–1																										15½–16 hrs	5 hrs
1–2																										15 hrs	4–4½ hrs
2–3																										14½ hrs	3½ hrs
3–4																										14½ hrs	3 hrs
4–6																										15 hrs	3 hrs
6–9																										14½–15 hrs	2½–3 hrs
9–12																										14½–15 hrs	2½–3 hrs

Daytime sleep
7:00 a.m.—7:00 p.m.

Nighttime sleep
7:00 p.m.—7:00 a.m.

Important Recommendations

The most recent advice from the Academy of American Pediatrics is that parents should allow their infants to room share, meaning sleep in their own bassinet or crib, in the room where their parents are. They recommend that the safest place for a baby to sleep is in a bassinet, crib or baby carrier, and that babies should be checked regularly when asleep. It is safest only to have bedclothes in the bed, and no objects such as toys or extra blankets. They also advise that a car seat is not an ideal place for infants to sleep in the home.

It is also important to remember that these recommendations are only for the first six months, and that after that time, you can start to settle your baby in his own room for naps and nighttime sleep. Until your baby reaches six months, you will have to alter the bedtime routine after his bath, so that you can finish off the remainder of the bedtime routine in the room where the baby is being settled to sleep for the evening. Replicate the same atmosphere in the living area as you would in the bedroom by keeping everything calm and quiet. It is unlikely that you will have a crib both upstairs and downstairs, therefore, according to the AAP, a bassinet with a proper mattress would be an acceptable option. (Throughout this book, in all routines up to six months, I refer to your baby's place of sleep as his "bed," which could be a bassinet, stroller or crib—or wherever he is settled to sleep.)

It is important to follow the same guidelines for settling your baby in the bassinet as those given for settling your baby in a crib. The baby should be placed in the bassinet with his feet at the bottom and it is essential that any sheets and blankets are tucked in securely so that they cannot work their way loose while he is sleeping.

◻ 6 ◻

Weeks One to Two

· · · · · · ·

· · · · · · · · ·
Starting the Routine

When moving on through the routines, it is important to remember that your baby's feeding and sleeping needs may not automatically fit straight into the feeding and sleeping times of the next routine. Don't start the next routine until your baby is following the routine he is in at present. However, some babies go through a stage of needing one routine for feeding but a different one for sleeping.

The following checklist will help you decide if your baby is ready to move on from feeding every three hours into the 1–2 week routine:

✳ Your baby has regained his birth weight.
✳ He is happily going three hours between feedings. The three hours are calculated from the beginning of one feeding to the beginning of the next feeding. This means that if a feeding has been taking

around one hour, there is only a two-hour gap between feedings.

✳ Your baby shows signs of wanting to go longer between some feedings—you have to wake him for some of his feedings.

✳ He is staying awake happily for a short time after some of his feedings.

If your baby is showing all of the above signs, you can confidently start to implement the 1–2 week routine. The 1–2 week routine is not so different to the every-three-hours routine, except that it starts to establish proper nap times, in particular the lunchtime nap. It is also when you start to introduce a proper bedtime routine and a longer sleep after the bedtime bath.

Your baby will still need to be fed every three hours during some parts of the day, but in the 1–2 week routine there is a split feeding at 10/11:15 a.m. in the morning, which helps establish the lunchtime nap. This routine also includes a split feeding at 5/6:15 p.m., which will help encourage a longer sleep between 7 p.m. and 10 p.m.

· · · · · · · · · · ·

Routine—1–2 Weeks

FEEDING TIMES	NAP TIMES BETWEEN 7 A.M. AND 7 P.M.
7 a.m.	8:30–10 a.m.
10 a.m.	11:30 a.m.–2 p.m.
11/11:15 a.m.	3:30–5 p.m.
2 p.m.	
5 p.m.	
6/6:15 p.m.	
10–11:15 p.m.	**Maximum daily sleep:** 5½ hours

Expressing times: 6:45 a.m. and 10:45 a.m.

· · · · · ·

7 A.M.

- ✳ Baby should be awake, diaper changed and fed with a bottle or breast no later than 7 a.m.
- ✳ He needs up to 25–35 minutes on the full breast; then offer 10–15 minutes on the breast from which you have expressed 3 oz.
- ✳ If he is fed at 5 a.m. or 6 a.m., offer up to 20–25 minutes from the second breast after expressing 3 oz.
- ✳ Do not feed baby after 8 a.m., as this will throw off his next feeding.
- ✳ He can stay awake for up to 1½ hours.
- ✳ Make sure you get some breakfast—have some cereal, toast and a drink no later than 8 a.m. while baby plays on his mat.

8:15 A.M.

- ✳ Baby should start to get a bit sleepy by this time. Even if he does not show the signs, he will be getting tired, so check his diaper and draw sheet and start winding down now.

8:30 A.M.

- ✳ When he is drowsy, settle baby in his bed, fully swaddled, no later than 8:30 a.m. He needs a nap of no longer than 1½ hours.
- ✳ Wash and sterilize any bottles and expressing equipment.

9:45 A.M.

- ✳ Unswaddle baby so that he can wake naturally.
- ✳ Prepare items for changing and dressing.

10 A.M.

 * Baby must be fully awake now, regardless of how long
   he slept.
 * He should be given up to 25–35 minutes from the breast
   he last fed on, while you drink a large glass of water.
 * Lay him on his play mat so that he can have a good
   kick, while you prepare equipment for expressing.

10:45 A.M.

 * Express 2 oz. from the second breast.
 * Wash (diaper area and face) and dress baby, remembering to cream all his creases and dry skin.

11/11:15 A.M.

 * Baby should start to get a bit sleepy by this time. Even
   if he does not show the signs, he will be getting tired,
   so check the draw sheet, change his diaper and start
   winding down now.
 * Offer baby up to 15–20 minutes from the breast you
   last expressed from.
 * When he is drowsy, settle baby in his bed, fully swaddled, no later than 11:30 a.m.
 * If he doesn't settle within 10 minutes, offer him up to
   10 minutes from the fuller breast. Do this with no
   talking or eye contact.

11:30 A.M.–2 P.M.

 * Baby needs a nap of no longer than 2½ hours from the
   time he went down.
 * If he wakes after 45 minutes, check the swaddle, but do
   not overstimulate him with lots of talking or eye contact.

✳ Allow 10 minutes for him to resettle himself; if he's still unsettled, offer him half his 2 p.m. feeding and settle him back to sleep until 2 p.m.

NOON

✳ Wash and sterilize expressing equipment, then you should have lunch and a rest before the next feeding.

2 P.M.

✳ Baby must be awake and feeding no later than 2 p.m., regardless of how long he has slept.

✳ Unswaddle him and allow him to wake naturally. Change his diaper.

✳ Give him up to 25–35 minutes from the breast he last fed on. If he is still hungry, offer up to 10–15 minutes from the other breast while you drink a large glass of water.

✳ Do not feed baby after 3:15 p.m. as it will throw off his next feeding.

✳ It is very important that he is fully awake now until 3:30 p.m., so he goes down well at 7 p.m.; if he was very alert in the morning, he may be sleepier now. Do not overdress him, as extra warmth will make him drowsy.

3:30 P.M.

✳ Change baby's diaper.

✳ Baby needs a nap of up to 1½ hours. This is a good time to take him for a walk to ensure that he naps well and is refreshed for his next feeding and bath.

✳ Baby should not sleep after 5 p.m. if you want him to go down well at 7 p.m.

5 P.M.

✳ Baby must be fully awake and feeding no later than 5 p.m.

✳ Give him up to 25–30 minutes from the breast he last fed on, while you drink a large glass of water.

✳ It is very important that he not doze while feeding and that he waits for the other breast until after his bath.

5:45 P.M.

✳ If baby has been very wakeful during the day or didn't nap well between 3:30 p.m. and 5 p.m., he may need to start his bath and next feeding early.

✳ Allow baby a good kick without his diaper while you prepare things needed for his bath and bedtime.

✳ Baby must start his bath no later than 5:45 p.m., and be massaged and dressed by 6/6:15 p.m.

6/6:15 P.M.

✳ Baby must be feeding no later than 6:15 p.m.; this should be done in a quiet, dimly lit room with care taken not to overstimulate him with lots of talking or eye contact.

✳ If he did not finish the first breast at 5 p.m., give him up to 5–10 minutes from it before putting him on the second breast. Allow up to 20–25 minutes from the second breast.

✳ It is very important that baby is in bed two hours from when he last woke.

7/7:15 P.M.

✳ When drowsy, settle baby in his bed, fully swaddled, no later than 7 p.m.

✳ If baby hasn't settled well, offer him up to 10 minutes from the fuller breast. Do this without overstimulating him with lots of talking or eye contact.

8 P.M.

✳ It is very important that you have a good meal and a rest before the next feeding.

9:45 P.M.

✳ Turn up the lights fully and unswaddle baby so that he can wake naturally. Allow at least 10 minutes before feeding to ensure that he is fully awake and can eat well.

✳ Lay out items for the diaper change, plus a spare draw sheet, burp cloth and receiving blanket in case they are needed in the middle of the night.

10 P.M.

✳ Give baby up to 25–35 minutes from the breast he last fed on, or most of his bottle-feeding, change his diaper and reswaddle him.

✳ Dim the lights and, with no talking or eye contact, give him up to 20–25 minutes on the second breast or the remainder of his bottle-feeding.

IN THE NIGHT

✳ During this week, it is important that breast-fed babies are not allowed to go too long in the night between feedings.

✳ A baby weighing less than 7 lbs. at birth should be woken at around 2:30 a.m. for a feeding, and a baby weighing 7–8 lbs. should be woken no later than 3:30 a.m.

✳ A formula-fed baby who weighs more than 8 lbs. or a baby that weighed more than 8 lbs. at birth, who has fed well during the day, may be able to go slightly longer, but not longer than five hours.

✳ If you are in doubt as to how long to allow your baby to sleep between feedings in the night, please seek advice from your pediatrician.

Changes to Be Made During the 1–2 Week Routine

Sleeping

Depending upon how long your baby sleeps after the late feeding, you can choose one of the following options:

✳ If your baby feeds well and settles well and then sleeps until after 2 a.m., then feeds well in the night and sleeps until closer to 6 a.m., following the routine and having him awake for an hour at the late feeding is fine.

✳ If your baby feeds well and settles well after being awake an hour at the late feeding, but then wakes before 2 a.m. and then wakes again before 6 a.m., I recommend splitting the late feeding to eliminate the twice-a-night waking. It can take at least a week to establish this split feeding so do not get disheartened if you do not see immediate results. For the split feeding to work well, you should start to wake your baby at around 9:45 p.m., and by 10 p.m. start the feeding. Give him as much as he wants, then allow him to play on his play mat. At close to 11 p.m. take him to the bedroom, change his diaper, then offer him the second part of his feeding. If he is formula-fed, I advise that you make two bottles.

Most babies in the early days can stay awake happily for up to two hours before needing a nap. This does not mean they must stay awake for the full two hours, only that it is important that they do not stay awake for longer if overtiredness is to be avoided. So if, during the early days, you find that your baby is only staying awake for 1–1½ hours at a time, you do not need to worry as he is obviously a baby that needs more sleep, and as he grows, he will start to stay awake longer.

Feeding

When your baby wakes in the night, it is important that he eats enough, so that he sleeps well until close to 6/7 a.m. You should not restrict the amount he wants to drink at this stage; by doing so you could risk him waking at 5 a.m. looking for another feeding. At this stage you are aiming to feed your baby well enough so that he only needs to feed twice between 7 p.m. and 6/7 a.m.

Depending upon what time he fed in the night, your baby will probably wake between 6 a.m. and 7 a.m., but he should always be woken at 7 a.m. If he wakes at 6 a.m., this means that you can give him most of his first morning feeding (treat this as a night feeding) and then offer him a top-up feeding at 7 a.m. He may then need a small feeding at 8:30 a.m. before his next nap.

During this routine I suggest that you always offer the baby a top-up feeding at 11/11:15 a.m., or just before the lunchtime nap. This will hopefully avoid him waking hungry during the middle of the nap. However, should he wake before 2 p.m., I would assume that hunger is the genuine cause and offer him a bottle or the breast before trying to settle him back to sleep. If he will not settle back to sleep, then it is best just to get him up, and then offer him two shorter naps at around 2:30 p.m. and 4/4:30 p.m.

Moving On to the 2–4 Week Routine

By the end of the second week, you should be able to advance on to the 2–4 week routine.

The following signs will help you decide whether your baby is ready to advance on to the 2–4 week routine.

* Your baby should weigh more than 7 lbs., have regained his birth weight and be gaining weight steadily.
* He is sleeping well at nap times and more often than not you have to wake him from his naps to feed him.
* He is feeding more efficiently and often finishing a breast within 25–30 minutes.
* He is showing signs of being more alert and managing to stay awake easily for 1½ hours at a time.

If you find that your baby is happy to go longer between feedings but still needs to sleep more than the 2–4 week routine suggests, then you can still follow this routine for feeding and continue to follow the 1–2 week routine for sleep until he shows signs of needing less sleep. Remember that a baby who needs more sleep will be sleeping well at night as well as during the day. If your baby is sleeping well during the day, but starting to be more wakeful in the middle of the night, it might be a sign that he needs to be awake more during the day.

7

Weeks Two to Four

· · · · · · ·

· · · · · · · ·
Routine—2–4 Weeks

FEEDING TIMES	NAP TIMES BETWEEN 7 A.M. AND 7 P.M.
7 a.m.	8:30/9–10 a.m.
10 a.m.	11:30 a.m./noon–2 p.m.
11:30/11:45 a.m.	4–5 p.m.
2 p.m.	
5 p.m.	
6/6:15 p.m.	
10–10:30 p.m.	**Maximum daily sleep:** 5 hours

Expressing times: 6:45 a.m., 10:30 a.m. and 9:30 p.m.

7 A.M.

✳ Baby should be awake, diaper changed and eating no later than 7 a.m.

✳ If he ate before 5 a.m., he needs up to 20–25 minutes from the full breast, then offer up to 10–15 minutes from the breast that you have expressed approximately 2–3 oz. from.

✳ If he fed at 5 a.m. or 6 a.m., offer up to 20–25 minutes from the second breast after expressing 3 oz.

✳ Do not feed baby after 7:45 a.m., as it will throw off his next feeding.

✳ He can stay awake for up to two hours.

✳ Have some cereal, toast and a drink no later than 8 a.m. while baby plays on his mat.

8:30/8:45 A.M.

✳ Baby should start to get a bit sleepy by this time. Even if he does not show the signs, he will be getting tired, so check his diaper and draw sheet and start winding down now.

✳ When he is drowsy, settle baby in his bed, fully swaddled, no later than 9 a.m. He needs a nap of no longer than 1½ hours.

✳ Wash and sterilize bottles and expressing equipment.

9:45 A.M.

✳ Unswaddle baby so that he can wake naturally.

✳ Prepare items for washing and dressing.

10 A.M.

✳ Baby must be fully awake now, regardless of how long he slept.

✳ He should be given up to 20–25 minutes from the breast he last fed on, while you drink a large glass of water.

✳ Wash and dress him, remembering to cream all his creases and dry skin.

10:30 A.M.

✳ Lay baby on his play mat so that he can have a good kick while you express 2 oz. from the second breast.

11:15/11:30 A.M.

✳ If baby was very alert and awake during the previous two hours, he may start to get tired by 11:15 a.m. and would need to be in bed by 11:30 a.m.

✳ Offer baby up to 15 minutes from the breast you last expressed from, immediately before going for his nap.

11:45 A.M.

✳ Regardless of what baby has done earlier, he should now be winding down for his nap.

✳ Check the draw sheet and change his diaper.

✳ When he is drowsy, settle baby in his bed, fully swaddled, no later than noon.

11:30 A.M./NOON–2 P.M.

✳ Baby needs a nap of no longer than 2½ hours from the time he goes down.

✳ If he slept 1½ hours earlier, only allow him two hours this nap time.

✳ If he wakes after 45 minutes, check the swaddle, but do not overstimulate him with lots of talking or eye contact.

✳ Allow 10–20 minutes for him to resettle himself; if he's still unsettled, offer him half his 2 p.m. feeding and settle him back to sleep until 2 p.m.

12/12:30 P.M.

✳ Wash and sterilize expressing equipment, then you should have lunch and a rest before the next feeding.

2 P.M.

＊ Baby must be awake and feeding no later than 2 p.m., regardless of how long he has slept.

＊ Unswaddle him and allow him to wake naturally. Change his diaper.

＊ Give him up to 20–25 minutes from the breast he last fed on. If he is still hungry, offer up to 10–15 minutes from the other breast, while you drink a large glass of water.

＊ Do not feed baby after 3:15 p.m. as it will throw off his next feeding.

＊ It is very important that he is fully awake now until 4 p.m., so he goes down well at 7 p.m.; if he was very alert in the morning, he may be sleepier now. Do not overdress him, as extra warmth will make him drowsy.

＊ Lay baby on his play mat and encourage him to move around.

3:45–4 P.M.

＊ Change baby's diaper.

＊ This is a good time to take him for a walk to ensure that he naps well, and is refreshed for his next feeding and bath.

＊ Baby should not sleep after 5 p.m. if you want him to go down well at 7 p.m.

5 P.M.

＊ Baby must be fully awake and feeding no later than 5 p.m.

＊ Give him up to 20 minutes from the breast he last fed on, while you drink a large glass of water.

＊ It is very important that he waits for the other breast until after his bath.

5:45 P.M.

✳ If baby has been very wakeful during the day, or didn't nap well between 4 p.m. and 5 p.m., he may need to start his bath and next feeding early.

✳ Allow baby a good kick without his diaper, while you prepare items needed for his bath and bedtime.

✳ Baby must start his bath no later than 6 p.m. and be massaged and dressed by 6:15 p.m.

6/6:15 P.M.

✳ Baby must be feeding no later than 6:15 p.m.; this should be done in a quiet, dimly lit room with care taken not to overstimulate him with lots of talking or eye contact.

✳ If he did not finish the first breast at 5 p.m., give him up to 5–10 minutes from it before putting him on the second breast. Allow up to 20–25 minutes from the second breast.

✳ It is very important that baby is in bed two hours from when he last woke.

7/7:15 P.M.

✳ When he is drowsy, settle baby in his bed, fully swaddled, no later than 7 p.m.

✳ If baby hasn't settled well, offer him up to 10–15 minutes from the fuller breast. Do this without overstimulating him with lots of talking or eye contact.

8 P.M.

✳ It is very important that you have a really good meal and a rest before the next feeding or expressing.

9:30 P.M.

✳ If you have chosen to replace the late feeding with a bottle-feeding, then express from both breasts now.

10/10:30 P.M.

✳ Turn up the lights fully and unswaddle baby so that he can wake naturally. Allow at least 10 minutes before feeding to ensure he is fully awake, so that he can nurse well.

✳ Lay out items for the diaper change, plus a spare draw sheet, burp cloth and receiving blanket in case they are needed in the middle of the night.

✳ Give baby up to 20 minutes from the breast he last fed on or most of his bottle-feeding, change his diaper and reswaddle him.

✳ Dim the lights and, with no talking or eye contact, give him up to 20 minutes from the second breast or the remainder of the bottle-feeding.

IN THE NIGHT

✳ If baby wakes before 4 a.m., it is important that you give him a big enough to drink to help him sleep closer to 7 a.m. If he falls asleep after feeding from one breast, and then he is waking again at 5 a.m., it is worth trying to get him slightly more awake so that he feeds from both breasts.

✳ If he wakes between 4 a.m. and 5 a.m., give him one breast, then start the 7 a.m. feeding on the fuller breast.

✳ If he wakes at 6 a.m., give him one breast and then the second at 7:30 a.m. after expressing.

✳ Keep the lights low and do not overstimulate him with lots of talking or eye contact. Only change his diaper if absolutely necessary or if he is too sleepy to take a full feeding.

· · · · · · · · · · ·

Changes to Be Made During the 2–4 Week Routine

The 2–4 week routine usually coincides with your baby's first growth spurt. Many babies become a bit fretful or unsettled during growth spurts, so arrange for your partner or another assistant to help with the bedtime routine. The majority of babies get a bit irritable around 5 p.m., and it is probably the most challenging time of the day for all mothers, so do not take it as a failure on your part if things get fraught at this time of the day.

Sleeping

By 3–4 weeks, your baby should start to show signs of being more awake and for longer periods. Ensure that you encourage the wakefulness during the day so that his nighttime sleep is not affected. By four weeks the morning nap should be no more than one hour, to ensure that he sleeps well at lunchtime.

Gradually, aim to keep him awake longer in the morning, until he is going down for his sleep at 9 a.m. If you find that he is going to sleep at 8:30 a.m. and waking between 9:15 a.m. and 9:30 a.m., which has an adverse effect on the rest of the day, giving him a head and face sponge bath around 8:20 a.m. is usually sufficient to revive him enough to last until 9 a.m. The afternoon nap should be no more than one hour in total; this nap is sometimes broken into a couple of catnaps between 4 p.m. and 5 p.m.

By five weeks, he should be half-swaddled, under the arms, for the morning and late-afternoon nap. Around four weeks, it becomes more obvious when the baby comes into his light sleep: normally every 45 minutes, although it can be every 30

· · · · · ·

minutes with some babies. If a feeding is not due, most babies, given the opportunity, settle themselves back to sleep. Rushing too quickly to your baby and assisting him back to sleep by rocking could result in a long-term sleep association problem. This means that in the night when your baby comes into his light sleep, you could end up getting up several times to help him back to sleep, long after the time he no longer needs night feedings.

Feeding

Most babies go through a growth spurt around the third week. When your baby goes through a growth spurt, reduce the amount you express at 6:45 a.m. by 1 oz. and by the end of the fourth week reduce the 10:30 a.m. expressing by 1 oz. This will ensure that your baby immediately receives the extra milk he needs. If you have not been expressing, you will need to allow your baby to feed more often on the breast and for longer periods, in order for him to get the amounts he needs. During this time, get extra rest so that your baby's increased feeding demands do not have the opposite effect on you, causing you to become so exhausted that your milk supply decreases even further. If you do not wish to lose his sleeping routine, you could try using the plan in Chapter Sixteen, Problem Solving in the First Year, which increases your milk supply without losing the sleep routine. Once your milk supply has increased, you can then go back to following the routine suitable for your baby's age.

Continuing to split the midmorning feeding and offering the baby a top-up of milk immediately before the lunchtime nap should help him sleep well here.

If you are breast-feeding and have decided to give one bottle-feeding a day, this is a good age to introduce it. If you leave it any later than this age, it is very possible that your baby will refuse a bottle altogether, which can cause enormous problems later on, particularly if you are going back to work. It is advisable to express between 9:30 p.m. and 10 p.m., extracting as much milk as possible, as this will help keep your milk supply up. This milk can either be used for the late feeding or frozen and used when you leave your baby with a babysitter. Introducing a bottle of expressed milk at the late feeding also allows your partner to get involved and enables you to get to bed earlier, giving you the extra sleep that all mothers need during the early weeks. If you wish to breast-feed for longer than six weeks, avoid giving formula at any other feedings, unless advised to do so by your doctor.

Bottle-fed babies should have their 7 a.m., 10 a.m. and late feedings increased first during growth spurts. Some bottle-fed babies are ready to go from using a newborn nipple to a slow-flow nipple.

A low milk supply or poor positioning at the breast usually causes low weight gain in breast-fed babies; the two often go hand in hand. It would be worthwhile following the plan for increasing your milk supply in Chapter Sixteen, Problem Solving in the First Year. I also advise that you arrange a home visit from a lactation consultant to check that you are positioning your baby on the breast correctly.

If your baby is formula-fed and not gaining sufficient weight, try moving him from the newborn nipple with one hole to the slow-flow nipple with two holes. Always discuss any concerns you have regarding your baby's low weight gain with your pediatrician.

If you find your baby is still waking at around 2 a.m. then again at 5 a.m., I would suggest that you introduce a split feeding at the late feeding. Start to wake him up at 9:45 p.m., so that he is wide awake by 10 p.m. Give him most of his feeding and keep him awake for longer than the recommended one hour. At 11:15 p.m. his diaper should be changed and the lights dimmed while you give him a small top-up feeding. By giving him a split feeding and having him awake slightly longer at this time, he will more than likely sleep well past 3 a.m., provided he is not getting out of his swaddle.

Once your baby reaches four weeks, he will probably show signs of being happy to go slightly longer between feedings, and you should be able to move him on to the four- to six-week feeding routine, provided he is gaining weight steadily. Babies who are not gaining sufficient weight should remain on the two- to four-week routine until their weight gain improves.

In my experience, babies who regularly gain between 6–8 oz. a week in the first few months are usually more content and sleep better than those who are putting on less than 6 oz. a week. On saying this, I have cared for some very happy and contented babies who would thrive well on a weight gain of only 4–5 oz. a week. However, if you find your baby is constantly irritable between feedings, not sleeping well at night and gaining less than 6 oz. a week, it may be that he is not getting enough to eat and it would be advisable to discuss his weight gain with your pediatrician.

8

Weeks Four to Six

• • • • • •

• • • • • • • • •
Routine—4–6 Weeks

FEEDING TIMES	NAP TIMES BETWEEN 7 A.M. AND 7 P.M.
7 a.m.	9 a.m.–10 a.m.
10:30 a.m.	11:30 a.m./noon–2/2:30 p.m.
2/2:30 p.m.	4:15 p.m.–5 p.m.
5 p.m.	
6/6:15 p.m.	
10/10:30 p.m.	**Maximum daily sleep:** 4¾ hours

Expressing times: 6:45 a.m., 10:30 a.m. and 9:30 p.m.

7 A.M.

❋ Baby should be awake, diaper changed and feeding no later than 7 a.m.

❋ If he fed before 5 a.m., he needs up to 20–25 minutes from the full breast. If he's still hungry, offer up to 10–15 minutes from the breast that you have expressed approximately 2 oz. from.

* If he fed at 5 a.m. or 6 a.m., offer up to 20–25 minutes from the second breast after expressing approximately 2 oz.
* Do not feed baby after 7:45 a.m., as it will throw off his next feeding.
* He can stay awake for up to two hours.
* Have some cereal, toast and a drink no later than 8 a.m. while baby has a kick on his play mat.

8:45 A.M.

* Baby should start to get a bit sleepy by this time. Even if he does not show the signs, he will be getting tired, so check his diaper and draw sheet and start winding down now.
* When he is drowsy, settle baby in his bed, fully or half-swaddled, no later than 9 a.m. He needs a nap of no longer than one hour.
* Wash and sterilize bottles and expressing equipment.

9:45 A.M.

* Unswaddle baby so that he can wake naturally.
* Prepare items for washing the baby's face and diaper area, and dressing.

10 A.M.

* Baby must be fully awake now, regardless of how long he slept.
* Wash and dress him, remembering to cream all his creases and dry skin.

10:30 A.M.

* Baby should be given up to 20–25 minutes from the breast he last fed on, while you drink a large glass of water.

✳ Lay him on his play mat so that he can have a good kick while you express 1 oz. from the second breast. Then offer him up to 10–15 minutes from this breast.

11:30 A.M.

✳ If baby was very alert and awake during the previous two hours, he may start to get tired by 11:30 a.m. and would need to be in bed by 11:45 a.m.

11:45 A.M.

✳ Regardless of what baby has done earlier, he should now be winding down for his nap.

✳ Check the draw sheet and change his diaper.

✳ When he is drowsy, settle baby in his bed, fully swaddled, no later than noon.

11:30 A.M./NOON–2/2:30 P.M.

✳ Baby needs a nap of no longer than 2½ hours from the time he went down.

✳ If he wakes after 45 minutes, check the swaddle, but do not overstimulate him with lots of talking or eye contact.

✳ Allow 10–20 minutes for him to resettle himself; if he's still unsettled, offer him half his 2 p.m. feeding and settle him back to sleep until 2 p.m.

NOON

✳ Wash and sterilize expressing equipment, then you should have lunch and a rest before the next feeding.

2/2:30 P.M.

✳ Baby must be awake and feeding no later than 2:30 p.m., regardless of how long he has slept.

✳ Unswaddle him and allow him to wake naturally. Change his diaper.

✳ Give him up to 20–25 minutes from the breast he last fed on. If he is still hungry, offer him up to 10–15 minutes from the other breast, while you drink a large glass of water.

✳ Do not feed baby after 3:15 p.m. as it will throw off his next feeding.

✳ It is very important that he is fully awake now until 4:15 p.m., so he goes down well at 7 p.m.; if he was very alert in the morning, he may be sleepier now. Do not over-dress him, as extra warmth will make him drowsy.

✳ Lay baby on his play mat and encourage him to kick his legs and move around.

4/4:15 P.M.

✳ Change baby's diaper.

✳ This is a good time to take him for a walk to ensure that he naps well and is refreshed for his next feeding and bath. He may start to cut back on this nap.

✳ Baby should not sleep after 5 p.m. if you want him to go down well at 7 p.m.

5 P.M.

✳ Baby must be fully awake and feeding no later than 5 p.m.

✳ Give him up to 20 minutes from the breast he last fed on, while you drink a large glass of water.

✳ It is very important that he waits for the other breast until after his bath.

5:45 P.M.

✳ If baby has been very wakeful during the day, or didn't

nap well between 4:15 p.m. and 5 p.m., he may need to start his bath and next meal early.

✳ Allow baby a good kick without his diaper while you prepare items needed for his bath and bedtime.

6 P.M.

✳ Baby must start his bath no later than 6 p.m. and be massaged and dressed by 6:15 p.m.

6:15 P.M.

✳ Baby must be feeding no later than 6:15 p.m.; this should be done in a quiet, dimly lit room with care taken not to overstimulate him with lots of talking or eye contact.

✳ If he did not finish the first breast at 5 p.m., give him up to 5–10 minutes from it before putting him on the second breast. Allow up to 20–25 minutes from the full breast.

✳ It is very important that baby is in bed two hours from when he last woke.

7 P.M.

✳ When he is drowsy, settle baby in his bed, fully swaddled, no later than 7 p.m.

✳ If baby hasn't settled well, offer him up to 10 minutes from the fuller breast. Do this without overstimulating him with lots of talking or eye contact.

8 P.M.

✳ It is very important that you have a good meal and a rest before the next feeding or expressing.

9:30 P.M.

✳ If you have chosen to replace the late breast-feeding with a bottle, then express from both breasts now.

10/10:30 P.M.

✳ Turn up the lights fully and unswaddle baby so that he can wake naturally. Allow at least 10 minutes before feeding to ensure that he is fully awake, so that he can eat well.

✳ Lay out items for the diaper change, plus a spare draw sheet, burp cloth and receiving blanket in case they are needed in the middle of the night.

✳ Give baby up to 20 minutes from the breast he last fed from or most of his bottle-feeding; change his diaper and reswaddle him.

✳ Dim the lights and, with no talking or eye contact, give him up to 20 minutes from the second breast or the remainder of the bottle-feeding.

IN THE NIGHT

✳ If baby wakes before 4 a.m., give him a full feeding.

✳ If he wakes between 4 a.m. and 5 a.m., give one breast, then start the 7 a.m. feeding on the fuller breast.

✳ If he wakes at 6 a.m., give him one breast, then the second at 7:30 a.m. after expressing.

✳ Keep the lights low and do not overstimulate him with lots of talking or eye contact. Only change his diaper if absolutely necessary or if he is too sleepy to eat a full amount.

· · · · · · · · · · · ·

Changes to Be Made During the 4–6 Week Routine

Sleeping

By the age of six weeks, the majority of babies that I cared for were sleeping for a much longer spell during the night, and many were sleeping through to closer to 7 a.m. Parents who are struggling to get their babies to sleep longer often ask me how I achieve this. My response has always been that by following the routines, it just happens naturally and that the babies themselves start to sleep longer and longer in the night. Certainly from reading the forums on my Web site, this seems to be true for the majority of parents. But what has also become obvious from reading thousands of posts over the last few years is that many of the parents whose babies do not manage by six weeks to sleep a longer stretch during the night appear to have much more sleep during the day than I recommend at this age. They believe that they have sleepy babies that need more daytime sleep. While I do believe that some babies need more sleep, from my personal experience those babies who genuinely needed more sleep would also begin to sleep longer in the night. If your baby is not showing signs of sleeping longer during the night, perhaps look more closely at his daytime sleep and gradually start to reduce the amount he is having. By putting him down for his first nap of the day a couple of minutes later every three or four days, it not only avoids the problem of him becoming overtired and not settling, it also reduces the amount of daytime sleep he gets.

I recommend that at this stage the daily nap time between 7 a.m. and 7 p.m. be reduced to a strict 4½ hours: the morning

· · · · · ·

nap should be no more than one hour, the afternoon nap no more than 30 minutes between 4:15 p.m. and 5 p.m. Some babies tend to doze off at around 8:30 a.m. and then sleep until closer to 10 a.m.; this results in too much daytime sleep and can affect how long the baby sleeps at night. If you find this is happening, I would suggest that you wake your baby at 9 a.m., so that he only sleeps 30 minutes; then allow him a further 15-minute catnap around 9:45 a.m. He should be fully awake by 10 a.m. This will keep his total morning sleep to just less than an hour, and by allowing only a 15-minute nap between 9:45 a.m. and 10:15 a.m., his lunchtime nap should not be affected.

It is very important that by the end of six weeks you start to get your baby used to being half-swaddled (under the arms) for the 9 a.m. and the 7 p.m. naps. Crib death rates peak between two and four months and overheating is considered to be a major factor in this. When you start to half-swaddle your baby, it is important to tuck him in securely. If he is waking earlier than the time the routine suggests, check if he has kicked his covers off; babies become more active at this age and this is another cause of them waking earlier in the night.

It should now take less time to settle your baby to sleep. The cuddling time should gradually be reduced. Now is a good time to get him used to going down when he is more awake. Often a lullaby light, which plays a tune and casts images on the ceiling for 10 minutes or so, will help a baby to settle himself.

Another important factor in helping your baby sleep longer in the night is to ensure that he is getting most of his daily milk intake between 6–7 a.m. and 11:30 p.m. A good indicator of this will be his weight gain; he should be gaining weight steadily. See the end of Chapter Seven, Weeks Two to Four, for information on weight gain.

Once he has slept a longer stretch several nights in a row, try not feeding him if he suddenly goes back to waking earlier again. The hours after the late feeding are sometimes referred to as the "core night" (see Chapter Sixteen, Problem Solving in the First Year, for a full explanation of the "core-night method").

On waking at this time, he should initially be left for a few minutes to settle back to sleep. If that doesn't work, use other methods to settle him. I would try giving him some cool boiled water or a cuddle; others recommend a pacifier. Attention should be kept to the minimum, while reassuring your baby that you are there. This teaches the baby one of the most important sleep skills: how to go back to sleep after surfacing from a non-REM sleep. Obviously, if he refuses to settle you would need to feed him. The core-night method can also be used to encourage an older baby who has gotten into the habit of waking at the same time in the night to sleep longer.

Before embarking on this method, the following points should be read carefully to make sure that your baby really is capable of going for a longer spell in the night:

* Never use these methods with a very small baby or a baby who is not gaining weight.
* These methods should only be used if your baby is gaining weight steadily and if you are sure that his last feeding is substantial enough to help him sleep for the longer stretch in the night.
* The main sign that a baby is ready to cut down on a night feeding is regular weight gain and the reluctance to feed or taking less at the 7 a.m. feeding.
* The aim of this method is gradually to increase the length of time your baby can go from his last feeding and not to eliminate the night feeding in one go. The

core-night method can be used if, over three or four nights, a baby has shown signs that he is capable of sleeping for a longer stretch. However, I cannot stress enough the importance of not using this method if your baby is not settling quickly in the night. If it is not working within three or four nights, you should abandon it and continue to feed your baby. If you persist with this method and your baby is not settling back quickly, you will actually create a sleep association problem that could mean your baby will continue to be unsettled in the night for many weeks.

Feeding

If your baby is feeding between 3 a.m. and 4 a.m., you have to wake him at 7 a.m. every morning for at least 10 days and he is starting to show less interest in his morning meal, then you can very gradually, and by a small amount, cut back the amount of milk he is taking in the night. This will have the domino effect of him drinking more during the day and less in the night, and eventually he will drop the middle-of-the-night feeding altogether. It is important not to cut back too much or too fast as the baby could then start to wake hungry long before 7 a.m.; this will defeat the whole purpose of getting him to sleep through from 11 p.m. to 6/7 a.m.

At around six weeks, your baby will go through another growth spurt, and you will need to reduce the amount you are expressing first thing in the morning by a further 1 oz. and cut out the midmorning expressing altogether. If your baby woke and fed well between 3 a.m. and 4 a.m., slept until 7 a.m., then woke and fed well again, he should be happy to go a stretch after the 7 a.m. feeding. You can gradually start to push the 10 a.m. feeding to closer to 10:30 a.m. The exception to this would be a baby who is feeding closer to 5 a.m. in the morning and having a top-up at 7:30 a.m. It is unlikely that he would get through to 10:30 a.m. if he's only had a top-up feeding at 7:30 a.m., so continue to feed him at 10 a.m. (with a top-up before the lunchtime nap) until he is feeding at between 6 a.m. and 7 a.m. During growth spurts, your baby will probably need to spend longer on the breast at some feedings, especially if you have not been expressing at the suggested times. It is important to allow the baby this extra time on the breast and, if need be, additional top-ups. While it may feel as if you are backtracking with the routines, the extra feeding during the day will only be short term and will avoid the problem of your baby starting to wake earlier or more in the night because he has not fed well enough during the day.

Bottle-fed babies should have the 7 a.m., the 10:30 a.m. and the 6:15 p.m. feedings increased first during growth spurts. If your baby is happily waiting until 10:30 a.m. for his feeding, and during this growth spurt, you find that he starts to wake during his lunchtime nap or earlier than usual, it would be worthwhile giving him a small top-up before putting him down for his nap. Once he has done a week of uninterrupted lunchtime naps, you can gradually cut back on the top-up until you have eliminated it altogether and he is back to having a full feeding at 10:30 a.m. However, should you find that your baby is more unsettled at the lunchtime nap without a top-up, there is no reason why you should not continue to offer it. The most important thing at this stage is that your baby sleeps well at the lunchtime nap.

9

Weeks Six to Eight

Routine—6–8 Weeks

FEEDING TIMES	NAP TIMES BETWEEN 7 A.M. AND 7 P.M.
7 a.m.	9 a.m.–9:45 a.m.
10:45 a.m.	11:45 a.m./noon–2/2:30 p.m.
2/2:30 p.m.	4:30 p.m.–5 p.m.
5 p.m.	
6/6:15 p.m.	
10/10:30 p.m.	**Maximum daily sleep:** 4 hours

Expressing times: 6:45 a.m. and 9:30 p.m.

7 A.M.

✳ Baby should be awake, diaper changed and eating no later than 7 a.m.

✳ If he fed before 5 a.m., he needs up to 20–25 minutes on the full breast. If he's still hungry, offer up to 10–15 minutes from the other breast after expressing 1–2 oz.

* If he ate at 6 a.m., offer him up to 20–25 minutes from the second breast after expressing 1–2 oz.
* Do not feed baby after 7:45 a.m., as it will throw off his next feeding.
* He can stay awake for up to two hours.
* Have some cereal, toast and a drink no later than 8 a.m. while your baby plays for a while on his play mat.
* Wash and dress baby, remembering to cream all his creases and dry skin.

8:50 A.M.

* Check baby's diaper and draw sheet and start winding down now.

9 A.M.

* Settle baby in his bed, half-swaddled, no later than 9 a.m. He needs a nap of no longer than 45 minutes.
* Wash and sterilize bottles and expressing equipment.

9:45 A.M.

* Unswaddle baby so that he can wake naturally.

10 A.M.

* Baby must be fully awake now, regardless of how long he slept.
* If baby ate a full amount at 7 a.m., he should last until 10:45 a.m. for his next feeding. If he ate earlier, followed by a top-up at 7:30 a.m., he may need to start this feeding slightly earlier.
* Encourage baby to play and kick his legs on his play mat.

10:45 A.M.

✳ Baby should be given up to 20–25 minutes from the breast he last fed on and then offered up to 10–15 minutes from the second breast, while you drink a large glass of water.

11:30 A.M.

✳ If baby was very alert and awake during the previous two hours, he may start to get tired by 11:30 a.m. and would need to be in bed by 11:45 a.m.

11:45 A.M.

✳ Regardless of what baby has done earlier, he should now be winding down for his nap.
✳ Check the draw sheet and change his diaper.
✳ Settle baby in his bed, half- or fully swaddled, no later than noon.

11:45 A.M./NOON–2/2:30 P.M.

✳ Baby needs a nap of no longer than 2½ hours from the time he went down.
✳ If he wakes after 45 minutes, check the swaddle, but do not overstimulate him with lots of talking or eye contact.
✳ Allow 10–20 minutes for him to settle himself; if he is still unsettled, offer him half his 2 p.m. feeding and settle him back to sleep until 2 p.m.

NOON

✳ Wash and sterilize expressing equipment if you didn't do this earlier; then you should have lunch and a rest before the next feeding.

2/2:30 P.M.

* Baby must be awake and feeding no later than 2:30 p.m., regardless of how long he has slept.
* Unswaddle him and allow him to wake naturally. Change his diaper.
* Give him up to 20–25 minutes from the breast he last fed on. If he is still hungry, offer him up to 10–15 minutes from the other breast, while you drink a large glass of water.
* Do not feed baby after 3:15 p.m. as it will throw off his next feeding.
* It is very important that he is fully awake now until 4:30 p.m., so he goes down well at 7 p.m.; if he was very alert in the morning, he may be sleepier now. Do not overdress him, as extra warmth will make him drowsy.
* Lay baby on his play mat for a while.

4:15/4:30 P.M.

* Change baby's diaper.
* This is a good time to take him for a walk to ensure that he naps well and is refreshed for his next meal and his bath.
* Baby should not sleep after 5 p.m. if you want him to go down well at 7 p.m.

5 P.M.

* Baby must be fully awake and eating no later than 5 p.m.
* Give him up to 20 minutes from the breast he last fed on, while you drink a large glass of water.
* It is very important that he waits for the other breast until after his bath.

5:45 P.M.

✳ If baby has been very wakeful during the day or didn't
nap well between 4:30 p.m. and 5 p.m., he may need to
start his bath and next feeding early.

✳ Allow baby a good kick without his diaper, while you
prepare items needed for his bath and bedtime.

6 P.M.

✳ Baby must start his bath no later than 6 p.m. and be
massaged and dressed by 6:15 p.m.

6:15 P.M.

✳ Baby must be feeding no later than 6:15 p.m.; this
should be done in a quiet, dimly lit room. Take care
not to overstimulate him with lots of talking or eye
contact.

✳ If he did not finish the first breast at 5 p.m., give him
up to 5–10 minutes from it before putting him on the
second breast.

✳ It is very important that baby is in bed two hours from
when he last woke.

7 P.M.

✳ Settle baby in his bed, half-swaddled, no later than 7 p.m.

8 P.M.

✳ It is very important that you have a good meal and a
rest before the next feeding or expressing.

9:30 P.M.

✳ If you have chosen to replace the late feeding with a
bottle-feeding, then express from both breasts now.

10/10:30 P.M.

❋ Turn up the lights fully and unswaddle baby so that he can wake naturally. Allow at least 10 minutes before feeding to ensure that he is fully awake, so that he can feed well.

❋ Lay out items for the diaper change, plus a spare draw sheet, burp cloth and receiving blanket in case they are needed in the middle of the night.

❋ Give baby up to 20 minutes from the breast he last fed on or most of his bottle-feeding; change his diaper and reswaddle him.

❋ Dim the lights and, with no talking or eye contact, give him up to 20 minutes from the second breast or the remainder of the bottle.

IN THE NIGHT

❋ If your baby is eating before 4 a.m. and losing interest in his 7 a.m. feeding, it would be wise to try settling him with some cool boiled water. If he even takes an ounce or two before going on the breast, it should have the domino effect of him eating better at 7 a.m. The aim is to get him to take all his daily requirements between 7 a.m. and 11 p.m. As long as he is gaining weight steadily, you can encourage him to cut down and eventually drop the night feeding. (See the core-night method in Chapter Sixteen, Problem Solving in the First Year.)

❋ If your baby becomes unsettled on being offered water, it is best to continue a little longer with a full feeding in the night.

❋ If he wakes at between 4 a.m. and 5 a.m., give one breast; then start the 7 a.m. feeding on the fuller breast.

✳ If he wakes at 6 a.m. give him one breast and then the second at 7:30 a.m. after expressing.

✳ Keep the lights low and do not overstimulate him with lots of talking or eye contact. Only change his diaper if absolutely necessary or if he is too sleepy to eat fully.

Changes to Be Made During the 6–8 Week Routine

Sleeping

Most babies who weigh more than 9 lbs. should be sleeping longer in the night now, provided they are getting most of their daily nutritional needs between 6–7 a.m. and 11 p.m. They should also be sleeping no more than four hours between 7 a.m. and 7 p.m. Once he has lasted longer for several nights in a row, try not feeding your baby before his latest time again. The morning nap should be no more than 45 minutes, the lunchtime nap should be 2¼–2½ hours—no longer—and the late-afternoon nap should be no more than 30 minutes. He may catnap on and off during this nap and some babies cut out this nap altogether. Do not allow him to cut out this nap if he is not managing to stay awake until 7 p.m. If you want him to sleep until 7 a.m., it is important that he goes to sleep closer to 7 p.m. Between six and eight weeks, you should ensure that your baby's morning nap is no longer than 45 minutes, as allowing longer than this could result in a shorter lunchtime nap. If you notice that your baby has already become more unsettled at lunchtime, despite offering a top-up before his nap, I would suggest cutting this nap to 30 minutes, even if it means bringing the time of the lunchtime nap forward slightly.

Lunchtime Nap

From six weeks onward, if your baby is sleeping the full 45 minutes in the morning, he should be woken after 2¼ hours. If for some reason his morning nap was much shorter, then you could allow him 2½ hours. If your baby develops a problem with his nighttime sleep, do not make the mistake of letting him sleep longer during the day. Keep his morning nap to no more than 30 minutes and his lunchtime nap to no more than 2 hours. It is at around eight weeks that the lunchtime nap may sometimes go wrong: you may find that your baby wakes 30–40 minutes after falling asleep and is unsettled. This is due to your baby taking on a more mature sleep cycle as he drifts from light sleep into a dreamlike sleep (known as REM) and then back into a deep sleep. While some babies only stir when they come into light sleep, others will wake fully. If your baby has not learned to settle himself and is consistently assisted back to sleep, then a real problem could develop. If he is waking during his lunchtime nap (and you are already offering a top-up before settling him), allow him 10–20 minutes to see if he will resettle himself. If he is unable to return to sleep or he becomes distressed at any point, go straight to him and offer him half of his 2 p.m. feeding (treated as a night feeding) before returning him to his bed. If he is still unsettled, just get him up for the afternoon.

Obviously, if his lunchtime nap was cut short, he cannot make it through from 1 p.m. to 4 p.m. happily. I find the best way to deal with this is to allow 30 minutes of nap time after the 2:30 p.m. feeding, then a further 20–30 minutes at 4:30 p.m. This should stop him getting overtired and irritable and get things back on track so that he goes to sleep well at 7 p.m. See Chapter Sixteen, Problem Solving in the First Year, for more in-depth solutions.

He should now be half-swaddled at the morning nap and 7 p.m. sleep and, by the end of eight weeks, also at the late feeding and in the night. Some babies may start to wake earlier in the night again once they are out of the swaddle; settle without feeding or reswaddling.

Feeding

During growth spurts, breast-fed babies should be given longer on the breast to ensure that their increased needs are met. If you have been expressing, you can reduce this by 1 oz. to ensure that his needs are immediately met and by the end of the eight weeks cut out the 6:45 a.m. expressing. If you have not expressed, you can still follow the feeding times from the routine for your baby's age, but you will have to top him up with a short breast-feed before his daytime naps. If you do this for a week or so, this should help increase your milk supply. A sign that this has happened is that your baby will sleep well at the naps and not be so interested in the next feeding. Once this happens you can gradually decrease the length of time that you top-up until you are back on your original feeding schedule. A formula-fed baby should have his feedings increased by 1 oz. when he is regularly draining his bottle, starting with the morning feeding. The late feeding should only be increased if all the other feedings have been increased and he is not going a longer spell in the night. Try not to give more than 6 oz. at this feeding unless your baby weighed more than 10 lbs. at birth. Some babies will need to move to a medium-flow nipple with three holes at this stage.

Between the ages of six to eight weeks, a baby who is gaining weight steadily and weighs more than 9 lbs. should be able to go longer from his late feeding—around five to six hours—provided he is eating well during the day and not sleeping more than the recommended amounts. If your baby is still waking between 2 a.m. and 3 a.m. despite drinking a good-sized amount, I advise, if you are not already doing so, that you give a split feeding at 10/11:15 p.m. The extra milk and time awake is often enough to help the baby sleep longer in the night. For this to work, it is important that you start to wake your baby no later than 9:45 p.m. so that he is fully awake and feeding by 10 p.m. Allow him to drink as much of the feeding as he would want, then put him on his play mat to exercise a bit. At 11 p.m. you should then take him to the bedroom and change his diaper; then offer him a further feeding. If you are formula-feeding, I advise that you make a fresh bottle for the second feeding.

If your baby then wakes in the night, check that he has not kicked off his covers, as this is another cause of nighttime waking in babies of this age. If he is securely tucked in but still waking, you should then settle him with some cool boiled water. If he refuses to settle, then you will have to feed him, but it would be advisable to refer to Chapter Four, Understanding Your Baby's Sleep, and Chapter Sixteen, Problem Solving in the First Year, to check for possible reasons why he is not sleeping for longer in the night. If he does settle, he will probably wake again around 5 a.m., at which time you can give him a full feeding, followed by a top-up at 7–7:30 a.m. This will help keep him on track with his feeding-and-sleeping pattern for the rest of the day.

Within a week, babies usually sleep until closer to 5 a.m., gradually increasing their sleep time until 7 a.m. Keep increasing day feedings, not night feedings. Most babies are happy to wait longer after the 7 a.m. feeding, so keep pushing this feeding forward until your baby is eating at 10:45 a.m. During this stage, when your baby is taking a top-up at 7–7:30 a.m. instead of a full feeding, he may not manage to get through to 10:45–11 a.m. for his next feeding. You may need to give him half a feeding at 10–10:15 a.m., followed by a top-up just before he goes down for his lunchtime nap, to ensure that he does not wake early from the nap. If your baby goes back to waking earlier again, wait 10 minutes or so before going to him. If he does not settle himself back to sleep, try settling him with some cool boiled water or a cuddle.

10

Weeks Eight to Twelve

· · · · · · ·

· · · · · · · ·
Routine—8–12 Weeks

FEEDING TIMES	NAP TIMES BETWEEN 7 A.M. AND 7 P.M.
7 a.m.	9 a.m.–9:45 a.m.
10:45/11 a.m.	noon–2/2:15 p.m.
2/2:15 p.m.	4:45 p.m.–5 p.m.
5 p.m.	
6/6:15 p.m.	
10/10:30 p.m.	**Maximum daily sleep:** 3½ hours

Expressing time: 9:30 p.m.

7 A.M.

✳ Baby should be awake, diaper changed and feeding no later than 7 a.m.

✳ He should be given up to 20 minutes from the first breast and then offered up to 10–15 minutes from the second breast.

* Do not feed baby after 7:45 a.m., as it will throw off his next feeding.
* He can stay awake for up to two hours.
* Have some cereal, toast and a drink no later than 8 a.m. while baby amuses himself on his play mat.
* Wash and dress baby, remembering to cream all his creases and dry skin.

8:50 A.M.

* Check baby's diaper and draw sheet.

9 A.M.

* Settle baby in his bed, half-swaddled, no later than 9 a.m. He needs a nap of no longer than 45 minutes.
* Wash and sterilize bottles and expressing equipment.

9:45 A.M.

* Unswaddle baby so that he can wake naturally.

10 A.M.

* Baby must be fully awake now, regardless of how long he slept.
* Encourage him to have fun on his play mat.

10:45/11 A.M.

* Baby should be given up to 20 minutes from the breast he last fed on and then offered up to 10–15 minutes from the second breast, while you drink a large glass of water.

11:45 A.M.

* Regardless of what baby has done earlier, he should now be winding down for his nap.

✳ Check the draw sheet and change his diaper.

✳ Settle baby in his bed, half-swaddled, no later than noon.

NOON–2/2:15 P.M.

✳ Baby needs a nap of no longer than 2¼ hours from the time he went down.

✳ If he wakes after 45 minutes, check the swaddle, but do not overstimulate him with lots of talking or eye contact.

✳ Allow 10–20 minutes for him to resettle himself; if he is still unsettled, offer him half of his 2 p.m. feeding and settle him back to sleep until 2/2:15 p.m.

✳ Wash and sterilize bottles and expressing equipment if you didn't do this earlier, then you should have lunch and a rest.

2/2:15 P.M.

✳ Baby must be awake 2¼ hours from the time he went down, regardless of how long he has slept, and he must be eating no later than 2:30 p.m.

✳ Unswaddle him and allow him to wake naturally. Change his diaper.

✳ Give him up to 20 minutes from the breast he last fed on. If he is still hungry, offer him up to 10–15 minutes from the other breast, while you drink a large glass of water.

✳ Do not feed baby after 3:15 p.m. as it will throw off his next feeding.

✳ It is very important that he is fully awake now until 4:45 p.m., so he goes down well at 7 p.m.

4:15 P.M.

* ✳ Change baby's diaper and offer him a small drink of cool boiled water no later than 4:30 p.m.
* ✳ He may have a short nap between 4:45 p.m. and 5 p.m.
* ✳ Baby should not sleep after 5 p.m. if you want him to go down well at 7 p.m.

5 P.M.

* ✳ Baby should be fully awake and feeding no later than 5 p.m.
* ✳ Give him up to 15 minutes from the breast he last fed on, while you drink a large glass of water.

5:45 P.M.

* ✳ If baby has been very wakeful during the day or didn't nap well between 4:45 p.m. and 5 p.m., he may need to start his bath and next feeding early.
* ✳ Allow baby a good kick without his diaper, while you prepare items needed for his bath and bedtime.

6 P.M.

* ✳ Baby must start his bath no later than 6 p.m. and be massaged and dressed by 6:15 p.m.

6:15 P.M.

* ✳ Baby must be eating no later than 6:15 p.m.; this should be done in a quiet, dimly lit room with care taken not to overstimulate him with lots of talking or eye contact.
* ✳ If he did not finish the first breast at 5 p.m., give him up to 5–10 minutes from it before putting him on the

second breast. Allow up to 20 minutes from the second breast.

✳ It is very important that baby is in bed two hours from when he last woke.

7 P.M.

✳ Settle baby in his bed, half-swaddled, no later than 7 p.m.

8 P.M.

✳ It is very important that you have a good meal and a rest before the next breast-feeding or expressing.

9:30 P.M.

✳ If you have chosen to replace the late nursing time with a bottle, then express from both breasts now.

10/10:30 P.M.

✳ Turn up the lights fully and unswaddle baby so that he can wake naturally. Allow at least 10 minutes before feeding to ensure that he is fully awake, so that he can eat well.

✳ Lay out items for the diaper change, plus a spare draw sheet, burp cloth and receiving blanket in case they are needed in the middle of the night.

✳ Give baby up to 20 minutes from the first breast or most of his bottle-feeding; change his diaper and re-swaddle him using a half swaddle.

✳ Dim the lights and, with no talking or eye contact, give him up to 20 minutes from the second breast or the remainder of the bottle-feeding.

IN THE NIGHT

✳ If your baby is nursing before 5 a.m., eating well and losing interest in his 7 a.m. meal, it would be wise to try settling him with some cool boiled water. Remember, the aim is to get him to take all his daily requirements between 7 a.m. and 11 p.m. As long as he is gaining weight steadily, he can be encouraged to go through to 7 a.m. without a milk feeding (see corenight method in Chapter Sixteen, Problem Solving in the First Year).

✳ If he wakes at 5 a.m., give him one breast and, if needed, 5–10 minutes from the second breast.

✳ If he wakes at 6 a.m., give him one breast and then the second at 7:30 a.m.

✳ Keep the lights low and do not overstimulate him with lots of talking or eye contact. Only change his diaper if absolutely necessary or if he is too sleepy to eat fully.

Changes to Be Made During the 8–12 Week Routine

Sleeping

Most babies who weigh close to 12 lbs. can manage to sleep through the night from the late feeding at this age, provided they are getting all of their daily nutritional needs between 7 a.m. and 11 p.m. They should also be sleeping no more than 3½ hours between 7 a.m. and 7 p.m. A totally breast-fed baby may still be waking once in the night, hopefully closer to 5 a.m. or 6 a.m.

Cut back your baby's daily nap time by a further 30 minutes, to a total of three hours. The morning nap should be no more than 45 minutes, but if he is not sleeping well at lunchtime, it can be cut back to 30 minutes. The lunchtime nap should be no more than 2¼ hours. It is around this stage that the lunchtime nap can sometimes go wrong. The baby comes into a light sleep usually 30–45 minutes after he has gone to sleep. Some babies will wake fully, and it is important that they learn how to settle themselves back to sleep to avoid the wrong sleep associations. For more details on this problem, refer to Chapter Sixteen, Problem Solving in the First Year.

Most babies have cut out their late-afternoon nap by now. If your baby hasn't, do not allow him to sleep for more than 15 minutes, unless for some reason the lunchtime nap has gone wrong, and then it should be slightly longer. All babies should only be half-swaddled, and particular attention should be paid when tucking in the baby.

One reason many babies of this age still wake in the night is because they move around the crib. If this is happening with your baby, you might purchase a light summer-weight sleeping bag. They are so lightweight that you can still use a sheet to tuck your baby in, without the worry of overheating.

Feeding

Your baby should be well established on five feedings a day now. If he is totally breast-fed and has started waking earlier in the morning, it may be worth trying a top-up from a bottle of either expressed or formula milk after the late feeding. If he is sleeping regularly until 7 a.m., gradually bring the late feeding forward by five minutes every three nights until he is feeding at 10 p.m. As long as he continues to sleep through to 7 a.m. and eats a full amount, you can keep pushing the 10:45 a.m. feeding back until it has become an 11 a.m. feeding.

Once your baby has slept through the night for two weeks, the 5 p.m. feeding can be dropped. I would not recommend dropping the split feeding until this happens, as a larger feeding at 6:15 p.m. could result in your baby taking even less at the last feeding, causing him to wake earlier in the morning. With many of the babies that I have cared for, I continued giving them a split feeding until solids were introduced to ensure that they were getting enough milk during the day. Once you eliminate the 5 p.m. feeding and your baby is taking a full feeding after his bath, he could cut down dramatically on his last feeding of the day, which could result in an early waking. If this happens, it is advisable to reintroduce a split feeding at 5–6:15 p.m. until your baby is fully established on solids and sleeping through to closer to 7 a.m.

If you are considering introducing a further bottle-feeding, the best time to introduce it is at the 11 a.m. feeding. Gradually reduce the time of this feeding by two or three minutes each day and top up with formula. By the end of the first week, if your baby is taking a 5–6–oz. bottle, you should be able to drop the breast-feed easily without the risk of serious engorgement. Bottle-fed babies should continue to have their 7 a.m., 11 a.m. and 6:15 p.m. feedings increased first during the next growth spurt at around nine weeks. Increase the amount of milk in the bottle-feeding to suit your baby's needs.

Moving on to the 3–4 Month Routine

As long as you are not exceeding your baby's daytime sleep and he is following the 8–12 week routine at night, then you can move on to the next routine. However, if, despite following all the advice, your baby is not sleeping as long in the night as the routine suggests, stick with this routine and try to improve the night sleeping. It might be worth dropping the late feeding for a short period to establish a longer period of sleep from 7 p.m. onward. Once a longer period of sleep becomes established, the late feeding can be reinstated, and hopefully, the baby's longer spell of sleep will then happen between 11 p.m. and 6/7 a.m. Once this happens, you can then move on to the 3–4 month routine.

11

Months Three to Four

· · · · · · ·

Routine—3–4 Months

FEEDING TIMES	NAP TIMES BETWEEN 7 A.M. AND 7 P.M.
7 a.m.	9–9:45 a.m.
11 a.m.	noon–2/2:15 p.m.
2:15/2:30 p.m.	
5 p.m.	
6/6:15 p.m.	
10/10:30 p.m.	**Maximum daily sleep:** 3 hours
Expressing time: 9:30 p.m.	

7 A.M.

⁎ Baby should be awake, diaper changed and eating no later than 7 a.m.

⁎ He should be given a full feeding from both breasts or from a bottle. By this stage, most babies reduce the amount of time they need to feed on the breast.

Be guided by your baby. If he is going happily from one feeding to the next, then he is likely getting enough milk.

✳ He can stay awake for around two hours.

8 A.M.

✳ Baby should be encouraged to amuse himself on his play mat for 20–30 minutes while you have breakfast.

✳ Wash and dress baby, remembering to cream all his creases and dry skin.

9 A.M.

✳ Settle baby in his bed, half-swaddled, no later than 9 a.m. He needs a nap of no longer than 45 minutes.

✳ Wash and sterilize bottles and expressing equipment.

9:45 A.M.

✳ Unswaddle baby so that he can wake naturally.

10 A.M.

✳ Baby must be fully awake now, regardless of how long he slept.

✳ Encourage him to kick on his play mat or take him on an outing.

11 A.M.

✳ Baby should be fed from both breasts or from a bottle.

11:50 A.M.

✳ Check the draw sheet and change his diaper.

✳ Settle baby, half-swaddled, no later than noon.

NOON–2/2:15 P.M.

* Baby needs a nap of no longer than 2¼ hours from the time he went down.

* Wash and sterilize bottles and expressing equipment if you didn't do this earlier; then you should have lunch and a rest before the next feeding.

2/2:15 P.M.

* Baby must be awake 2¼ hours from the time he went down, regardless of how long he has slept, and he must be eating no later than 2:30 p.m.

* Unswaddle him and allow him to wake naturally. Change his diaper.

* He should be allowed to drink from both breasts or from a bottle.

* Do not feed baby after 3:15 p.m. as it will throw off his next feeding.

* If he has slept well at both naps, he should manage to get through the rest of the afternoon without sleeping any more.

4/4:15 P.M.

* Change baby's diaper and offer him a drink of cool boiled water no later than 4:30 p.m.

* If he did not sleep well at lunchtime, he may need a short nap sometime between 4:30 p.m. and 5 p.m.

* Baby should not sleep after 5 p.m. if you want him to go down well at 7 p.m.

5 P.M.

* Give him up to 15 minutes from the breast he last fed on or from a bottle.

5:45 P.M.

❋ Allow baby a good kick without his diaper, while you prepare items needed for his bath and bedtime.

6 P.M.

❋ Baby must start his bath no later than 6 p.m. and be massaged and dressed by 6:15 p.m.

6:15 P.M.

❋ Baby must be eating no later than 6:15 p.m.

❋ If he did not finish the first breast at 5 p.m., give him up to 5–10 minutes from it before putting him on the second breast. Allow him up to 20 minutes from the second breast or a bottle.

❋ Dim the lights and sit baby in his chair for 10 minutes while you tidy up.

7 P.M.

❋ Settle baby in his bed, half-swaddled, no later than 7 p.m.

8 P.M.

❋ It is very important that you have a good meal and a rest before the next feeding or expressing.

9:30 P.M.

❋ If you have chosen to replace the late feeding with a bottle, then express from both breasts now.

10/10:30 P.M.

❋ Turn up the lights and unswaddle baby so that he can wake naturally.

✳ Give him most of his breast-feed or bottle, change his diaper and half-swaddle him.

✳ Dim the lights and, with no talking or eye contact, give him the remainder of his feeding.

. . . .

Changes to Be Made During the 3–4 Month Routine

Sleeping

If you have structured the milk feedings and nap times according to the routine, your baby should manage to sleep through the night from the late feeding to close to 6–7 a.m. in the morning. If he shows signs of starting to wake earlier, assume that it may be due to hunger. Increase his late feeding and, if need be, go back to offering a split feeding at this time. You should also ensure that his maximum daily sleep between 7 a.m. and 7 p.m. totals no more than three hours. Some babies may need less sleep than this, and you may have to look at cutting his total daytime sleep back to around 2½ hours, with a 30-minute nap in the morning and a two-hour nap at lunchtime.

If your baby is following the routine well, he will have cut back on his late-afternoon nap. On some days, he may manage to get through the afternoon without the nap but may need to go to bed five to 10 minutes earlier on those days. Should your baby have slept less than two hours at lunchtime, he should certainly be encouraged to have a short nap of no longer than 30 minutes between 4 p.m. and 5 p.m., otherwise he may become so overtired at bedtime that he doesn't settle to sleep easily.

Between three and four months, the time that your baby is awake at the late feeding should be gradually reduced to 30 minutes, provided he has been sleeping through regularly to 7 a.m., for at least two weeks. This should be very quiet and treated like a middle-of-the-night feeding. Bring it forward by 10 minutes every three nights until it becomes a very quick, sleepy feeding at 10 p.m. However, if your baby is still waking at between 5 a.m. and 6 a.m., it would be advisable to continue to keep him awake for at least an hour at the late feeding, making it a split feed.

Even if he is not getting out of his half-swaddle, I suggest that now is a good time to get him used to a 100 percent cotton, very lightweight sleeping bag. He will still need to be tucked in firmly, with one sheet, and perhaps one blanket, depending upon the room temperature; therefore, it is important the sleeping bag is light to avoid the risk of overheating.

Feeding

Between three and four months, if your baby has slept through the night until 7 a.m. for at least two weeks, you should ensure that any extra milk needed during growth spurts is increased at daytime feedings to prevent him backtracking on his nighttime waking. If your baby is totally breast-fed and is still waking in the night despite being topped up with expressed milk at the late feeding, it could be that he will need more to drink at this time. If you are unable to express extra milk earlier in the day, some mothers find that topping up with a small amount of formula at this feeding helps. You should discuss this with your doctor.

If your baby is formula-fed 7–8 oz. four times a day, he may only need 4–6 oz. at the late feeding. However, if your baby is not sleeping through the night at this age, it may be because he needs a little extra at this feeding.

Even if it means he cuts back on his morning feeding, I suggest offering him a full feeding of 7–8 oz. for several nights to see if that will help him sleep for longer in the night.

Some babies simply refuse the late feeding at three to four months. However, if you find that he starts to wake earlier again and will not settle back to sleep within 10 minutes or so, you should assume that he's hungry and should feed him. You may then have to consider reintroducing the late feeding until he is weaned and established on solids.

If you find that your baby keeps on waking before 4/5 a.m., refuses cool boiled water and will not settle without feeding, keep a very detailed diary listing exact times and amounts of feeding and times of daytime naps to try to determine whether the waking is habit or actual hunger.

Whether you are breast- or bottle-feeding, if your baby's weight gain is good, you are convinced he is waking from habit and he refuses cool boiled water, try waiting 15–20 minutes before going to him. Some babies will actually settle themselves back to sleep. A baby of this age may still be waking in the night because he is getting out of his covers. Tuck him in tightly.

If your baby is formula-fed and is taking 35–40 oz. of formula between 7 a.m. and 11 p.m., he should not really need to eat during the night. However, some very big babies who weigh more than 15 lbs. at this stage may still need to feed between 5 a.m. and 6 a.m., followed by a top-up at 7–7:30 a.m. until they reach six months and are weaned. Current guidelines are that babies should not be weaned before six months. If you are concerned that your baby is showing all the signs of needing to be weaned (see Chapter Fifteen, Introducing Solid Food), it is important that you discuss this with your pediatrician.

It is better to keep feeding in the night for a slightly longer time than to take the risk of weaning your baby before he is ready. A totally breast-fed baby may also need to feed at around 5–6 a.m. as he may not be getting enough to eat at the last feeding. A good indicator of whether your baby is ready to drop the night feeding—regardless of whether he is breast- or bottle-fed—is how he takes his top-up at 7–7:30 a.m. If he takes it greedily, he is probably genuinely hungry at 5–6 a.m. If he fusses and frets and refuses the top-up, I would assume the early wakeup is more habit than hunger; try to settle him back with some cool boiled water or a cuddle.

If your baby continues to sleep through to 7 a.m. once his waking time at the late feeding has been reduced to 30 minutes, plus he is cutting back on his 7 a.m. feeding, start very slowly reducing the amount he is drinking at the late feeding. Only continue with this if he is sleeping well until 7 a.m. However, I would not advise dropping this feeding altogether until he reaches six months and solids have been established. If you abandon the late feeding before solids are introduced, and your baby goes through a growth spurt, you may find that you have to go back to feeding him in the middle of the night.

If your baby is exclusively breast-fed and weighs more than 14 lbs., you may find that during growth spurts you have to go back to feeding him in the middle of the night, until solids are introduced. If you feel that your milk supply is low, follow the plan for increasing milk supply in Chapter Sixteen, Problem Solving in the First Year.

12

Months Four to Six

· · · · · ·

········

Routine—4–6 Months

FEEDING TIMES	NAP TIMES BETWEEN 7 A.M. AND 7 P.M.
7 a.m.	9–9:45 a.m.
11 a.m.	noon–2/2:15 p.m.
2:15/2:30 p.m.	
6/6:15 p.m.	
10 p.m.	**Maximum daily sleep:** 3 hours

Expressing time: 9:30 p.m.

7 A.M.

* Baby should be awake, diaper changed and eating no later than 7 a.m.
* He should be given a full feeding from both breasts or from a bottle.
* He can stay awake for around two hours.

8 A.M.

✳ Baby should be encouraged to amuse himself on his play mat or enjoy other activities for 20–30 minutes while you have breakfast.

✳ Wash and dress baby, remembering to cream all his creases and dry skin.

9/9:15 A.M.

✳ Settle baby in his sleeping bag, securely tucked in, no later than 9:15 a.m. He needs a nap of 30–45 minutes.

✳ Wash and sterilize bottles and expressing equipment.

9:45 A.M.

✳ Untuck him so that he can wake naturally.

10 A.M.

✳ Baby must be fully awake now, regardless of how long he slept.

✳ Encourage him to exercise on his play mat or take him on an outing.

11 A.M.

✳ Baby should be given a feeding from both breasts or from a bottle before being offered solids if you have been advised to wean early.

✳ Encourage him to sit in his chair while you clear away the lunch things.

11:50 A.M.

✳ Check the draw sheet and change his diaper.

✳ Settle baby in his sleeping bag, securely tucked in, no later than noon.

NOON

* Baby needs a nap of no longer than 2¼ hours from the time he went down.
* You should have lunch and a rest before the next feeding.

2/2:15 P.M.

* Baby must be awake 2¼ hours from the time he went down, regardless of how long he has slept, and he must be eating no later than 2:30 p.m.
* Untuck baby and allow him to wake naturally. Change his diaper.
* He should be given a feeding from both breasts or from a bottle.
* Do not feed baby after 3:15 p.m. as it will throw off his next feeding.
* If he has slept well at both naps, he should manage to get through the rest of the afternoon without further sleep.

4:15 P.M.

* Change baby's diaper and offer him a drink of cool boiled water no later than 4:30 p.m.
* If he did not sleep well at lunchtime, he may need a short nap sometime between 4:30 and 5 p.m.
* Baby should not sleep after 5 p.m. if you want him to go down well at 7 p.m.

5 P.M.

* By now, baby should be happy to wait to eat until after his bath. If not, offer him up to 10–15 minutes from the breast he last fed on or from a bottle.

5:30 P.M.

＊ Allow baby a good kick without his diaper, while you prepare items needed for his bath and bedtime.

5:45 P.M.

＊ Baby must start his bath no later than 5:45 p.m. and be massaged and dressed between 6 p.m. and 6:15 p.m.

6/6:15 P.M.

＊ Baby should start to eat between 6 p.m. and 6:15 p.m., depending upon how tired he is.

＊ He should be given a full feeding from both breasts or from a full bottle. If he ate at 5 p.m. but did not finish the first breast, give him up to 5–10 minutes from it before putting him on the second breast. Allow him up to 20 minutes from the second breast or a bottle.

＊ Dim the lights and sit baby in his chair for 10 minutes while you tidy up.

＊ If you have been advised to wean baby early, offer him his solids now.

7 P.M.

＊ Settle baby in his sleeping bag, securely tucked in, no later than 7 p.m.

＊ It is very important that you have a good meal and a rest before the next feeding or expressing.

9:30 P.M.

＊ If you have chosen to replace the late feeding with a bottle, then express from both breasts now.

10 P.M.

✳ Turn up the lights and wake baby enough to eat.

✳ Remove his sleeping bag, give him most of the feeding, change his diaper and then replace his sleeping bag.

✳ Dim the lights and, with no talking or eye contact, give him the remainder of the feeding. If he does not want the remainder, do not force it; he could start to cut back on this feeding now.

✳ This feeding should take no longer than 30 minutes.

✳ Tuck baby in securely with a thin sheet.

Changes to Be Made During the 4–6 Month Routine

Sleeping

Between four and six months, your baby should manage to sleep from the late feeding until 6/7 a.m. in the morning, provided he is taking 4–5 full milk feedings a day, and not sleeping more than three hours between 7 a.m. and 7 p.m.

If he is still waking in the night and you are confident that it is not due to hunger, I would advise trying the core-night method, as described in Chapter Sixteen, Problem Solving in the First Year. If this does not work, it could be that your baby needs less sleep, and I would suggest gradually cutting back on his daytime sleep to 2½ hours. If after a couple of weeks this has not improved things, then I would suggest dropping the late feeding to see how long he will sleep. The time he wakes will help you decide whether to continue with the late feeding. For example, if he sleeps until 5 a.m., then eats and settles back to sleep until 7 a.m., he will at least be sleeping one longer spell between

7 p.m. and 7 a.m., and this would be preferable to him waking and feeding at both the late feeding and at 5 a.m.

However, if you drop the feeding and he wakes at something like 1 a.m. and 5 a.m., then it would make sense to continue with the late feeding so that he doesn't wake and eat twice between midnight and 5 a.m.

If your baby weighs more than 15 lbs., genuine hunger could be the cause of night waking, particularly if he is fully breast-fed. If this is the case, then you may have to accept that he will need to nurse during the night until he is established on solids at six months. If you feel that he is showing signs that he is ready to be weaned, consult your pediatrician for advice as to whether he should begin earlier than the recommended six months. If you decide to continue to feed him in the middle of the night, it is crucial to ensure that he is fed quickly and quietly and that he settles back into a sound sleep until 7 a.m.

If you have not already introduced a sleeping bag, I advise doing so at this stage. If you leave it any later, he may be unhappy about being put into one.

Until your baby is able to crawl and maneuver himself around the crib, he still needs to be tucked in firmly. In very hot weather he can be put into a very light cotton sleeping bag, with just a diaper on, and tucked in with a very thin crib sheet.

If he is not sleeping the full two hours at lunchtime, cut back his morning nap to 20–30 minutes, and then bring the 11 a.m. feeding forward to 10:30 a.m. Top him up with some milk just before he goes down for his lunchtime nap.

Feeding

I recommend that you continue to offer your baby the late feeding until solids are introduced. The Academy of American Pediatrics recommends that solids be introduced between four and six months. As your baby will continue to go through growth spurts between four and six months, his nutritional needs will still need to be met. In my experience, this can rarely be done on four milk feedings a day. If you decide to drop the late feeding and he starts to wake earlier and not settle back to sleep quickly, then you should assume that it is hunger and feed him. It would then be worth considering reintroducing the late feeding until solids are established. If you find that he refuses a late feeding, but wakes at 5 a.m. hungry, then you should feed him and settle him back to sleep until 7 a.m., then offer him a top-up feeding before 8 a.m. If this happens, you may then have to feed him earlier, between 10 a.m. and 10:30 a.m., but then I suggest that you offer him a further top-up before he goes down for his lunchtime nap to ensure that he sleeps well.

During growth spurts, you may find that your baby is not content on five feedings a day. If this is the case, you may have to offer a split feeding in the morning and reintroduce the 5 p.m. feeding if you had previously dropped it.

If your baby becomes very discontented between feedings, despite being offered extra milk, and you think that he is showing signs of needing to be weaned, then it is important to discuss this with your doctor. If weaning your baby before six months is recommended, introduce solids very carefully. Solids should only be seen as tasters at this stage and given in addition to milk; they should not be a replacement. To ensure this does not happen, always make sure that your baby drinks all his milk first. Start with a small amount of baby rice mixed with either breast milk or formula after the 11 a.m. feeding. Once he is taking this, you can then transfer the rice to after the 6 p.m. feeding and start to introduce some of the first weaning foods recommended in Chapter Fifteen, Introducing Solid Food after the 11 a.m. feeding.

If you find that your baby is too tired to take all of his milk at 6 p.m. followed by the solids, give him two-thirds of the milk at 5:15/5:30 p.m., followed by the solids and followed by the remainder of his milk after bath time. If you are formula-feeding, it is advisable to make two separate bottles to ensure that the milk is fresh.

Once solids are introduced at this feeding, and as they increase, your baby should automatically cut back on his late feeding. Once he is down to taking only a very short breast-feed or just a couple of ounces of formula at the late feeding and continuing to sleep well through to 7 a.m., you should be able to drop the late feeding without risking that he will wake earlier in the morning.

A breast-fed baby who has reached five months, is weaned and is now starting to wake before 10 p.m., may not be getting enough at this time. Try giving a full breast-feed at 5:30 p.m. followed by the solids, with a bath at 6:15 p.m., followed by a top-up of expressed milk or formula after the bath. A baby who is not weaned would more than likely need to continue to have a split-milk feeding at 5/6:15 p.m. until solids are introduced.

13

Months Six to Nine

· · · · · ·

Once your baby is six months old, it is time for him to sleep in his own room. Because he will be used to always having people around him during nap times and in the evening, it is best to do this gradually. Start by settling him at either the morning or lunchtime nap in his own room. Once he is sleeping well at either of these times, you can then move on to settling him in his own room from 7 p.m. As your baby will not have been used to sleeping in the dark for daytime naps, I suggest that you allow him a small night-light for naps and at bedtime, until he is more accustomed to sleeping in his own room. Gradually phase this out once he is settling and sleeping well at these times.

Routine—6–9 Months

FEEDING TIMES	NAP TIMES BETWEEN 7 A.M. AND 7 P.M.
7 a.m.	9:15/9:30–10 a.m.
11:30 a.m.	12:30–2:30 p.m.
2:30 p.m.	
5 p.m.	
6:30 p.m.	**Maximum daily sleep:** 2½–2¾ hours

7 A.M.

✳ Baby should be awake, diaper changed and eating no later than 7 a.m.

✳ He should be given a full feeding from both breasts or from a bottle, followed by breakfast cereal mixed with either expressed milk or formula and fruit, once weaning is established.

✳ He can stay awake for 2–2½ hours.

8 A.M.

✳ Baby should be encouraged to play on the floor or enjoy other activities for 20–30 minutes while you have breakfast.

✳ Wash and dress baby, remembering to cream all his creases and dry skin.

9:15/9:30 A.M.

✳ Close the curtains and settle baby in his sleeping bag—in the dark with the door shut—no later than 9:30 a.m. He needs a nap of 30–45 minutes.

9:55 A.M.

✳ Open the curtains and undo his sleeping bag so that he can wake naturally.

✳ Baby must be fully awake by 10 a.m., regardless of how long he slept.

✳ Encourage him to play on the floor or take him on an outing.

11:30 A.M.

✳ By seven months, baby should be given most of his solids before being offered a drink of water or well-diluted juice from a cup, then alternate between solids and a drink.

✳ Encourage him to sit in his chair with some finger foods while you have lunch.

✳ Keep pushing the time of your baby's lunch later until it is closer to midday.

12:20 P.M.

✳ Check the draw sheet and change his diaper.

✳ Close the curtains and settle baby, in his sleeping bag—in the dark with the door shut—no later than 12:30 p.m.

12:30–2:30 P.M.

✳ Baby needs a nap of no longer than two hours from the time he goes down.

2:30 P.M.

✳ Baby must be awake and eating no later than 2:30 p.m., regardless of how long he has slept.

* Open the curtains and undo his sleeping bag so that he can wake naturally. Change his diaper.
* He should be nursed from both breasts or given a bottle.
* Do not feed baby after 3:15 p.m. as it will throw off his next feeding.

4:15 P.M.

* Change baby's diaper.

5 P.M.

* Baby should be given most of his solids before being offered a small drink of water from a cup. It is important that he still has a good milk feeding at bedtime, so keep this drink to a minimum.

6 P.M.

* He must start his bath no later than 6 p.m. and be massaged and dressed by 6:30 p.m.

6:30 P.M.

* Baby must be eating no later than 6:30 p.m. He should be nursed from both breasts or given a bottle.
* Dim the lights and read him a story.

7 P.M.

* Settle baby in his sleeping bag—in the dark with the door shut—no later than 7 p.m.

· · · · · · · · · · ·

Changes to Be Made During the 6–9 Month Routine

Sleeping

Once your baby is established on three meals a day, he should manage to sleep from around 7 p.m. to 7 a.m. The sooner you wean him off milk and onto solid food (4–6 months being the Academy of American Pediatrics recommended range), the less likely he will still need a small late feeding.

If your baby is not cutting down on his late feeding once solids are established, he is probably either not getting the right quantities of solids for his age or weight, or he needs a bigger feeding at 6:30 p.m. Keep a diary of all food and milk consumed over a period of four days to help pinpoint why he is not cutting out that last feeding. If you are confident that his food intake is sufficient and he is taking the late feeding from habit rather than from genuine hunger, gradually start to reduce it. If you reduce it by an ounce every three to four days, provided he does not start to wake early, continue to do this until he is taking only a couple of ounces. Once he is taking a couple of ounces, you can then drop it altogether so he can sleep straight through from 7 p.m. to 7 a.m.

Once he reaches six months, aim to keep pushing the morning nap forward to 9:30 a.m., and encourage him to go down for his lunchtime nap closer to 12:30 p.m. This is important once solids are established and he is having three full meals a day, with lunch coming around 11:45 a.m./noon. Some babies are happy to sleep later in the morning once they are established on three meals a day. If your baby sleeps until closer to 8 a.m., he will not need a morning nap but may not manage to

· · · · · ·

get through until 12:30 p.m. for his lunchtime nap; therefore, he may need to have lunch around 11:30 a.m. so he can go down at 12:15 p.m. for his lunchtime nap (see Chapter Sixteen, Problem Solving in the First Year).

Between six and nine months, your baby will start to roll onto his front and may prefer to sleep on his tummy. When this happens, I suggest you remove the sheet and blanket to avoid him getting tangled in them. In the winter months, the lightweight sleeping bag will need to be replaced with a warmer one to make up for the loss of blankets.

Feeding

If you have waited until six months to introduce solids, it is important that you work through the different foods fairly quickly and keep increasing the amounts every couple of days or when your baby shows signs of wanting more. Start by introducing baby rice after the 11 a.m. feeding, and then every couple of days introduce a new food, from the first-stage foods.

Once your baby is taking a reasonable amount of solids at lunch, you can introduce solids at breakfast. As your baby approaches seven months, he should be ready to drop his 11 a.m. milk feeding and have protein introduced at lunchtime.

If you were advised to wean your baby early, you will probably have worked your way through the list of first-stage weaning foods by the time he reaches six months. Once he is taking around six tablespoonfuls of mixed vegetables at lunchtime, you can then introduce the second-stage foods, which include protein.

For more information on the first and second stages of weaning see Chapter Fifteen, Introducing Solid Food.

By the end of six months, your baby will probably be ready

to sit in a high chair for his meals. Always ensure that he is properly strapped in and never left unattended.

It is important that you introduce your baby to a cup at lunchtime between the ages of six and seven months and that you start to use the tier system of feeding at that time. Once your baby is only taking a couple of ounces of milk at lunch, replace it with a drink of water or well-diluted juice from a cup. It is important that this is done once your baby is eating protein at lunchtime. Once the milk is dropped, he may need to increase the 2:30 p.m. feeding. However, if you do that and then notice that he is cutting back too much on his last feeding, continue to keep this feeding smaller.

Between six and seven months, solids should be transferred and changed to a solid late-afternoon snack at 5 p.m. with only a small drink of water from a cup, if you have not already done this. He would then have a full milk feeding around 6:30 p.m.

By nine months, if your baby is formula-fed, he should be drinking all of his water, diluted juice and most of his milk from a cup.

It is important to begin to clean your baby's teeth as soon as the first one appears. At this stage you will probably find it easiest to use a small piece of clean gauze wrapped around your finger, along with a small amount of special baby toothpaste, which can be massaged all around the baby's gums and teeth. Later, when more teeth have appeared, you can move on to a soft baby toothbrush for cleaning.

14

Months Nine to Twelve

· · · · · · ·

Routine—9–12 Months

FEEDING TIMES	NAP TIMES BETWEEN 7 A.M. AND 7 P.M.
7 a.m.	9:30–10 a.m.
11:45 a.m./noon	12:30–2:30 p.m.
2:30 p.m.	
5 p.m.	
6:30 p.m.	**Maximum daily sleep:** 2–2½ hours

7 A.M.

* Baby should be awake, diaper changed and eating no later than 7 a.m.
* He should be nursed from both breasts or given formula from a cup, followed by breakfast cereal mixed with expressed milk or formula, fruit and finger foods.
* He can stay awake for at least 2½ hours.

8 A.M.

✳ Baby should be encouraged to play on the floor or enjoy other activities for 20–30 minutes while you have breakfast.

✳ Wash and dress baby, remembering to cream all his creases and dry skin.

9:30 A.M.

✳ Close the curtains and settle baby in his sleeping bag—in the dark with the door shut—at around 9:30 a.m. He needs a nap of 15–30 minutes.

9:55 A.M.

✳ Open the curtains and undo his sleeping bag so that he can wake naturally.

✳ Baby must be fully awake by 10 a.m., regardless of how long he slept.

✳ Encourage him to play on the floor or take him on an outing.

11:45 A.M./NOON

✳ Baby should be given most of his solids before being offered a drink of water or well-diluted juice from a cup; then alternate between solids and a drink.

✳ Encourage him to sit in his chair with some finger foods, while you have lunch.

12:20 P.M.

✳ Check the draw sheet and change his diaper.

✳ Close the curtains and settle baby in his sleeping bag—in the dark with the door shut—no later than 12:30 p.m.

✳ He needs a nap of no longer than two hours from the time he goes down.

2:30 P.M.

✳ Baby must be awake and eating no later than 2:30 p.m., regardless of how long he has slept.

✳ Open the curtains, and undo his sleeping bag so that he can wake naturally. Change his diaper.

✳ He should be nursed or given a cup of formula, water or well-diluted juice, and perhaps a snack if he no longer has milk at this time.

✳ Do not feed baby after 3:15 p.m. as it will throw off his next feeding.

4:15 P.M.

✳ Change baby's diaper.

5 P.M.

✳ Baby should be given most of his solids before being offered a small drink of water or milk from a cup. It is important that he still has a good milk feeding at bedtime, so keep this drink to a minimum.

6 P.M.

✳ He must start his bath no later than 6 p.m. and be massaged and dressed by 6:30 p.m.

6:30 P.M.

✳ Baby should be eating no later than 6:30 p.m.

✳ He should nurse from both breasts or have 7–8 oz. of formula; this will eventually be reduced to 5–6 oz. when a cup is introduced at one year.

❋ Dim the lights and read him a story.

7 P.M.

❋ Settle baby in his sleeping bag—in the dark with the door shut—no later than 7 p.m.

. . . .

Changes to Be Made During the 9–12 Month Routine

Sleeping

At this stage, most babies cut back significantly on their daily sleep. If you notice that your baby is starting to wake in the night or earlier in the morning, you should cut back on the amount of sleep he is getting during the day.

The first nap to cut back on is the morning one. If that has been 30 minutes long, then try cutting it back to 10–15 minutes. Some babies may also cut back their lunchtime nap to 1½ hours, which can lead to them becoming very tired and irritable in the late afternoon. If this happens to your baby, try cutting out the morning nap altogether to see if it improves his lunchtime sleep. You may have to make lunchtime slightly earlier if he can't make it through to 12:30 p.m. for his nap.

Your baby may also start to pull himself up in the crib but get very upset when he can't get himself back down. If this happens, I suggest you encourage him to practice lying down when you put him down for his naps. Until he is able to maneuver himself up and down, you will need to help him settle back down. It is important that you do so with the least amount of fuss and talking. It is also worth taking a look at his daytime sleep total, as waking and standing up in the night can be a

. . . . . .

product of too much daytime sleep, which is easily rectified by cutting down, or cutting out, the morning nap. Some babies who cut out their morning nap earlier than the average will start to eliminate their lunchtime nap at this stage. It is not unheard of for a baby 1½ months old to need a nap of only an hour or so (between 1 and 2 p.m.) and still sleep soundly until 7 a.m.

Feeding

Your baby should be well established on three meals a day, and should also be able to feed himself some of the time. It is very important that your baby learns to chew properly at this stage. Most of his meals should consist of foods that have been chopped, sliced or diced. By the end of his first year, he should be able to manage chopped meat. This is also a good time to introduce raw vegetables and salads. Include some finger foods at every meal. If he shows an interest in holding his own spoon, do not discourage these attempts. It is important that he enjoys his food—even if a certain amount of it lands on the floor.

At nine months, a formula-fed baby should be taking all of his water, diluted juice, breakfast milk and 2:30 p.m. feeding from a cup. By the age of one year, he should be drinking all fluids from a cup.

For more information on solid food at this stage, see Chapter Fifteen, Introducing Solid Food.

15

Introducing Solid Food

Weaning Your Baby

The latest recommendations from the American Academy of Pediatrics advise that breast milk or formula be your child's sole source of nutrition for the first 4–6 months and the major source of nutrition throughout the first twelve. This is because it takes up to four months for the lining of a baby's stomach to develop and for the kidneys to mature enough to cope with the waste products from solid foods. If solids are introduced before a baby has the complete set of enzymes required to digest food properly, his digestive system could be damaged. Many experts blame the rapid increase in allergies over the last 20 years on babies being weaned before their digestive system is ready to cope.

During the writing of the latest edition of this book, I spoke to many dietitians and pediatricians as well as hundreds of mothers via my Web site. It is clear that there is some controversy surrounding these recommendations. Certainly, there are health professionals who feel that introducing solid foods between four and six months is not what threatens a baby's health, but the kinds of food the baby is given. It is also clear that many babies cannot manage on milk alone for the full six months. I urge you to discuss any and all of your concerns with your doctors and to follow their advice accordingly.

The golden rules: Do not give your baby solid food before 17 weeks. Do not begin weaning before neuromuscular coordination has developed sufficiently so that the baby can control his head and neck while sitting upright supported in a chair to be fed. He should also be able to swallow food easily by moving it from the front of his mouth to the back.

If you follow the weaning plan in this book and introduce the recommended foods in the order suggested, you can be confident that you are not putting your baby at risk of food allergies. Babies rely on the introduction of iron-containing foods at six months as that is when their bodies' iron stores with which they are born become depleted. Iron is essential for healthy red blood cells that transport oxygen around the body. Children who do not take in sufficient amounts of iron are at risk of developing iron-deficiency anemia, which causes tiredness, irritability and an overall lack of energy and enthusiasm. Once a baby has been weaned off the breast or bottle entirely, do not hesitate to introduce iron-containing foods, such as breakfast cereals, broccoli, lentils and baby foods fortified with iron. You will need to progress quickly through the food groups to include meat or vegetarian alternatives for their iron content. Babies on formula will have their iron supplemented in the milk.

I do not know your baby and cannot tell you when he is ready to be weaned. All babies should be watched closely for signs that they are ready for weaning, which might possibly come sooner than the AAP recommendations. If your baby is less than six months old and showing all the signs of being ready to wean, it is vital you discuss the situation with your doctors and decide with them whether to wean early.

I hope the following guidelines will help you identify possible signs of being ready to wean.

* He has been taking a full feeding four or five times a day from both breasts or an 8-oz. bottle of formula and has been happily going for four hours between feedings but now gets irritable and chews his hands long before his next feeding is due.
* He has been taking a full feeding from both breasts or an 8-oz. bottle of formula and screams for more the minute the milk is gone.
* He usually sleeps well at night and nap times but is starting to wake earlier and earlier.
* He is chewing his hands excessively, displaying eye-to-hand coordination and trying to put things into his mouth.

If your baby is more than four months old, has doubled his birth weight and is consistently displaying most of these signs, he could be ready to begin weaning. If the baby is less than six months old, you should tell your pediatrician and decide how to proceed. If you decide to wait until the baby is six months before you introduce solids, it is important that his increased hunger is met by increased amounts of milk feedings. Babies who have been sleeping through the night with only a small feeding at 10:30 p.m. would need to have this feeding increased. And, if they go through a further growth spurt before they reach six months, it may be that you need to introduce a further feeding in the middle of the night. It is very important to understand that as your baby grows, so will his appetite. If you wish to continue exclusive breast-feeding until six months, it is unreasonable to expect the baby to manage on only four milk feedings a day.

Breast-fed Babies

With babies who are being breast-fed exclusively, it is more difficult to tell how much milk they are receiving. If your baby is more than four months and showing most of the signs in the previous Weaning Your Baby section, you will need to talk to your doctor about the choices available to you.

If he is less than four months and not gaining enough weight each week, it is possible that your milk supply is getting too low in the evening. All that may be needed is extra milk. I suggest you try topping up the baby with a couple of ounces of expressed or formula milk after the late feeding. If this does not work or if he is waking more than once in the night, I would replace the late feeding altogether with a full bottle if you have not already done so. Encourage your partner to offer this feeding so that you can get to bed after expressing whatever milk you have between 9:30 and 10 p.m. to avoid your supply falling any further. Mothers in this situation often find that when they express they are only producing 3–4 oz., which is much less than their baby may need at this feeding. The expressed milk can be given at some other feeding during the day, thus avoiding further complementary bottle-feeding.

This plan usually satisfies a baby's hunger and improves his weight gain. You should never wean a baby before 17 weeks of age, and if sooner than six months, it should be done only in consultation with your pediatrician.

. . . .

Foods to Be Avoided

During the first two years of your baby's life certain foods are best used sparingly or avoided altogether as they may be harmful to your baby's health. The two worst culprits in this regard are sugar and salt.

Sugar

During the first year of weaning, it is best to avoid adding sugar to any of your baby's food, as it may cause him to develop a taste for sweet things. A baby's appetite for savory foods can be seriously affected if he is allowed lots of food containing sugar or sugar substitutes. These ingredients can be hard to avoid in commercially prepared food. When choosing baby cereals or commercial foods, check the labels carefully; sugar may be listed as dextrose, fructose, glucose or sucrose. Watch out, too, for syrup or concentrated fruit juice, which is also sometimes used as sweeteners.

Too much sugar in the diet can also lead to serious problems such as tooth decay and obesity. Because sugar converts very quickly into energy, babies and children who have too much may become hyperactive. Products such as baked beans, cornflakes, fish sticks, jam, tomato ketchup, canned soups and some yogurts are just a few of the everyday foods that contain hidden sugars. The American Academy of Pediatrics recommends that fruit juice not be given to babies less than six months and to limit the amount given to babies and toddlers to 4–6 oz. a day.

. . . . . .

Salt

Children less than two years old should not have salt added to their food—they get all the salt they need from natural sources such as vegetables. Adding salt to a young baby's food can be very dangerous, as it may put a strain on his immature kidneys. Research also shows that children with high salt intake may be more prone to heart disease later. When your baby reaches the stage of joining in with family meals, it is important that you do not add salt to the food during cooking. Remove your baby's portion, then add salt if needed for the rest of the family.

As with sugar, many processed foods and commercially prepared meals contain high levels of salt. It is important to check the labels on these foods carefully before giving them to your toddler.

Honey

Children should not eat honey until they are 12 months old. Younger than that, their digestive systems can not handle the spores of a common bacteria found in honey that are harmless to older children and adults. Honey can make children younger than one year old seriously, even fatally, ill.

. . . .

Preparing and Cooking Food for Your Baby

Making your own food can be more cost effective and will be of great nutritional benefit for your baby. You can save time and effort by making large quantities at a time and storing mini meals in the freezer. Keep sterilized feeding equipment, ice cube trays and freezer-proof containers at the ready and follow these general instructions:

✳ When preparing food, always ensure that all surfaces are clean and have been wiped down with an anti-bacterial cleaner. Use paper towels for cleaning surfaces and drying as they are more hygienic than kitchen cloths and towels.

✳ All fresh fruit and vegetables should be rinsed thoroughly with filtered water, then carefully peeled, removing the core, seeds and any blemishes.

✳ If you are advised to wean your baby early, remember that all fruits and vegetables must be cooked until your baby is six months old. This can be done by either steaming or boiling them in filtered water. Do not add salt, sugar or honey.

✳ During the initial stages of weaning, all food must be cooked until it is soft enough to puree to a very smooth consistency. A small amount of the cooking water may be added so that the mixture is similar to smooth yogurt.

✳ If using a food processor, check carefully for lumps by using a spoon and pouring into another bowl. Then transfer to ice cube trays or containers for storage in the freezer.

Sterilized Feeding Equipment

All feeding equipment should be sterilized for the first six months and bottles and nipples for as long as they are used. Sterilize ice cube trays or freezer containers by boiling them in a large saucepan of water for five minutes. Use a steam sterilizer, if you have one, for small items such as spoons and serving bowls, and follow timings recommended in the manufacturer's handbook. Wash cooking utensils as usual in a dishwasher or rinse hand-washed items with boiling water from a kettle.

Packing Food for the Freezer

* Make sure cooked, pureed food is covered as quickly as possible and transferred into the freezer as soon as it is cool enough.
* Never put warm food into a refrigerator or freezer.
* Check the temperature of your freezer with a freezer thermometer. It should read −18°C. Freezer thermometers can be purchased from a good hardware store or the cookware section of a large department store.
* If using an ice cube tray, fill with pureed food, open-freeze until solid, then pop the cubes out of the tray and into a sterilized plastic box. Non-sterilized items such as plastic bags can be used once the baby is six months old. Seal well and freeze.
* Label items clearly, including the date.
* Use foods within six months.
* Never refreeze cooked food. Food can only be put back into the freezer if it was originally frozen raw and then defrosted and cooked—a raw frozen chicken breast, defrosted, for example, can be frozen as a cooked casserole.

Defrosting Tips

* Defrost frozen (covered) food in the fridge overnight or leave at room temperature for short periods if you forget, transferring it into the fridge within a couple hours. Make sure it is covered at all times and placed on a plate to catch the drips.
* Never speed up defrosting by putting food into warm or hot water.
* Always use defrosted foods within 24 hours.

Reheating Tips

- Food should be heated thoroughly to ensure that any bacteria are killed. If food was frozen in jars, always transfer it into a dish; never serve it straight from the jar. Any food left over should be discarded, never reheated and used again. Babies are much more susceptible to food poisoning than adults are, so get in the habit of throwing leftovers away immediately.
- When batch cooking, take out a portion of food for your baby to eat now and freeze the rest. Don't be tempted to reheat the entire mixture and then freeze what is left.
- If your baby has eaten only a tiny portion, it can be tempting to reheat and serve leftovers later. Do not do so.
- Reheat food only once.

Early Weaning

If you have been advised that your baby is ready for weaning before the recommended age of six months, remember that milk is still the most important food for him. It provides him with the right balance of vitamins and minerals. Solids given before six months are classed as first tastes and fillers, which should be increased very slowly over several weeks, gradually preparing your baby for three solid meals a day. By offering the milk first, you will ensure that his daily milk intake is adequate for his nutritional needs.

Remember that as soon as your baby has teeth and has begun on any type of solid food, he will need his teeth cleaned twice a day, preferably after each meal.

How to Begin

✳ Introduce solids after the 11 a.m. feeding. Prepare everything you need for giving the solids in advance: a baby chair, bib, spoon, bowl and a clean, fresh damp cloth.

✳ Start by offering your baby a teaspoonful of pure rice mixed to a very smooth consistency using either expressed milk, formula or cool, filtered freshly boiled water.

✳ Make sure the rice has cooled enough before feeding it to your baby. Use a shallow plastic spoon for him— never a metal one, which can be too sharp or get too hot.

✳ Some babies need help in learning how to eat from the spoon. By placing the spoon just far enough into his mouth, and bringing the spoon up and out against the roof of his mouth, his upper gums will take the food off, encouraging him to eat.

✳ Once your baby is established on baby rice at 11 a.m. and is tolerating it, give the rice after the 6 p.m. feeding instead. When he finishes the one teaspoonful and shows signs of looking for more food, the amount of solids can be increased, provided he continues to take the required amount of milk at 6 p.m.

✳ Once your baby is happily taking 1–2 teaspoonfuls of baby rice mixed with milk or water after the 6 p.m. feeding, a small amount of pear puree can be introduced after the 11 a.m. meal. With babies less than six months old, this usually happens between the fourth and sixth day, and with babies more than six months it will probably happen between the second and fourth day.

✳ Be guided by your baby as to when to increase the amounts. He will turn his head away and get fussy when he has had enough.

✳ If the baby tolerates the pear puree, transfer it to the 6 p.m. meal. Mixing the puree with baby rice in the evening will make it more palatable and prevent your baby from becoming constipated.

✳ Small amounts of various organic vegetables and fruit can now be introduced, one by one, after the 11 a.m. meal. To prevent your baby from developing a sweet tooth, give more vegetables than fruit. At this stage, avoid the stronger-tasting ones such as spinach or broccoli, but rather concentrate on root vegetables (such as carrots, sweet potatoes and turnips). These contain natural sugars, will taste sweeter and blander, and may prove more palatable to your baby.

✳ With babies less than six months old, it is important to introduce new foods in small amounts and every 3–4 days. Increasing 1–2 teaspoonfuls a week between the two meals is a good guideline. Babies more than six months will probably need their meals increased by larger amounts every couple of days, and as long as you stick to the foods listed in first-stage weaning, you can introduce new foods closer together. Keeping a food diary will help you see how your baby reacts to each new food.

✳ Always be very positive and smile when offering a new food even if your baby spits it out; it may not mean he dislikes it. Remember this is all very new to him and different foods will get a different reaction. If he positively refuses a food, however, leave it and try again a week later.

✳ Always offer milk first, as nutritionally this is still the most important food at this stage. While appetites do vary, in my experience, the majority of babies are still drinking four to five full servings of formula or breast milk a day. Provided your baby is happy and thriving, the minimum daily recommended amount of milk required at this age, once solids are established, is 20 oz. a day.

. . . .

First Stage: 6–7 Months

If your baby started solid foods before six months, he will probably have tasted baby rice, plus a variety of different vegetables and fruits. If not, follow my guidelines (in this chapter) for when to start baby on rice and when to introduce fruit and vegetables. Once you have started weaning, it is important to keep introducing a variety of the different fruits and vegetables listed in the first-stage foods. All fruit and vegetables should still be steamed or cooked in filtered water until soft, then pureed. Mix to the desired consistency with some of the cooking water, or no-salt chicken stock may be used with some vegetables.

You should avoid introducing dairy products, wheat, eggs, nuts and citrus fruit as they are the foods most likely to trigger allergies. Honey should not be introduced before one year. Meat, chicken and fish should not be introduced until the babies are capable of digesting reasonable amounts of other solids. Some nutritionists believe that protein can put a strain on the young baby's kidneys and digestive tract. I agree. All too often I have seen feeding problems occur because meat, poultry or fish have been introduced too early. Once you have worked

. . . . . .

through the first foods, you can introduce protein. In the meantime, your first sources of iron can be found in lentils, broccoli and iron-rich breakfast cereals.

If you begin weaning at the age of six months, you will need to progress quickly through the first-stage foods so the iron-rich meat and vegetarian products can be introduced regularly. A rough guideline would be to increase the baby rice at the 5 p.m. meal by one teaspoonful every couple of days. It is also essential to rapidly reduce your baby's milk intake to four feedings a day once solids are established.

Between six and seven months, depending upon when you began weaning, your baby should be having 2–3 servings of carbohydrates daily in the form of cereal, whole wheat bread, pasta or potatoes. He should also have three servings of vegetables or fruit each day and one serving of animal or vegetable protein.

Foods to Introduce

Pure baby rice, pear, apple, carrot, sweet potatoes, potatoes, green beans, and zucchini are ideal first weaning foods. Once your baby is happily taking these foods, you can introduce parsnips, mango, peaches, broccoli, avocados, barley, peas and cauliflower.

Protein in the form of beef, poultry, fish and lentils should be introduced between six and seven months, once your baby is taking a reasonable amount of solids. Check that all the bones are removed and trim off the fat and the skin. Some babies find the flavor of protein cooked on its own too strong. Try cooking chicken or beef in a casserole with familiar root vegetables and fish in a milk sauce until your baby becomes accustomed to the different texture and taste. Cook meat with vegetables as a casserole and pulse in a food processor.

Start introducing protein at lunchtime as it is harder to digest than carbohydrates and will be digested by bedtime.

Introducing Breakfast

A baby is ready to start having breakfast once he shows signs of hunger long before his 11 a.m. meal. This usually happens between the ages of six and seven months. Once your baby is eating breakfast, you can gradually start to move the 11 a.m. feeding later, eventually settling somewhere between 11:30 a.m. and noon. I find that organic rice or millet cereal with a small amount of pureed fruit is a favorite with most babies. By seven months, if your baby is eating a full breakfast of cereal, fruit and perhaps small pieces of toast, you should aim to cut back the amount offered to him from the bottle. Give part of the milk as a drink and the remainder with the cereal. Always encourage your baby to take at least 5–6 oz. before giving him solids.

If you are still breast-feeding, gradually reduce the time your baby is on the first breast, then give him his solids and, finally, a further short feeding from the second breast. Be very careful not to increase his solids so much that he cuts back too much on his breast-feeding.

If your baby reaches seven months and is refusing breakfast, you can always cut back his milk slightly to encourage him to take small amounts of solids.

Regardless of whether you introduced solids before six months or at six months, aim to have a feeding plan similar to the one below before you introduce protein. This will ensure that your baby's system can cope.

7/7:30 a.m.	Breast-feed or 6–8 oz. of formula
	2–3 teaspoons of oat cereal mixed with breast milk or formula and 1–2 tablespoons of fruit puree
11:15/11:30 a.m.	Breast-feed or 2–3 oz. of formula
	2–3 tablespoons of sweet potato puree and 2–3 tablespoons of root vegetable puree plus 1–2 tablespoons of cauliflower or green vegetable puree mixed with some chicken stock
2/2:30 p.m.	Breast-feed or give 5–7 oz. formula
6 p.m.	Breast-feed or give 6–8 oz. of formula
	5–6 teaspoons of baby rice mixed with breast milk, formula or cool boiled water, then mixed with 2 tablespoons of fruit puree

Introducing Protein at Lunchtime

Once your baby is eating around six cubes or tablespoons of mixed vegetables, you should be able to introduce protein foods. If you started weaning your baby at six months, it could take between two to three weeks for him to be taking that amount. The best way to introduce the protein is to start by replacing two of the vegetables with two servings of chicken, red lentils or fish. Introduce new protein foods slowly at this stage—one every three days is about right. If your baby has no reaction, then keep replacing one or two tablespoons of vegetables every day until the complete serving of vegetables is replaced with a complete serving of protein.

Once your baby is taking a full protein meal at lunchtime, it is important to introduce him to a cup with a drink of water or well-diluted juice. Between the ages of six and seven months, you should start to use the tier system of feeding during that meal. Start this once your baby starts to take no more than a couple of ounces of milk. Once the lunchtime milk is dropped, he may need to drink more during the 2:30 p.m. feeding. However, if you notice that he is cutting back too much on his 5 p.m. afternoon snack or bedtime feeding, continue to keep this feeding smaller.

Once protein meals are established at lunchtime, give your baby a solid snack at 5 p.m., with only a small drink of water from a cup. Then, at around 6:30 p.m., give a full milk feeding.

Introducing a Cup

Once protein is well established, your baby's milk feeding should be replaced at lunchtime by a drink of cool boiled water or well-diluted juice from a cup. Most babies are capable of sipping and swallowing at this age, and this behavior should be encouraged by always offering the lunchtime drink from a cup. Do not worry if your baby only drinks a small amount at this meal. You will probably find that he makes up for it at his 2:30 p.m. feeding or takes an increase of cool boiled water later in the day. If you find that your baby's sleeping becomes unsettled at lunchtime when you drop the milk feeding, you may for a short time have to go back to offering him a small top-up of milk before the lunchtime nap, but it is important that you keep persevering with offering him fluids from his cup at lunchtime.

Late-afternoon Snack

Once you feel confident that the lunchtime solids are going well, you can then replace the cereal and fruit given after 6 p.m. with a solid snack, which I developed in England to coincide with late afternoon. If you always make sure that your baby has a well-balanced breakfast and lunch, you can be relaxed about this meal. Once breakfast and lunch are established, you can sit the baby down at 5 p.m. and offer him a late-afternoon snack. Some babies can get very fractious around this time of the day, so offer foods that are quick and easy to prepare—thick vegetable soups and vegetables that have been prepared and frozen in advance are always a good standby. Pasta, or a baked potato, served with vegetables and a sauce is also nutritious and easy. A very hungry baby can also be offered a custard or yogurt. Once you provide this, follow it at 6:30 with a full bottle.

Daily Requirements

By now, your baby will probably be eating two solid meals a day. Now it is important that you work toward establishing your baby on three proper meals per day. Each of these should include three servings of carbohydrates, such as cereals, bread and pasta, plus at least three servings of vegetables and fruit, and one serving of pureed meat or fish or two servings of beans and peas. By six months, a baby has used up most of the iron stores with which he was born. Because his iron requirements between six and twelve months are particularly high, it is important that his diet provides the right amount of this mineral. To help iron absorption in cereals and meat, always serve them with fruit or vegetables rich in vitamin C.

Getting the right balance of solids is vital so that he continues to get the right amount of milk. Although he will already have cut down on the 11 a.m. breast- or bottle-feeding of milk as his intake of solids increases, he still needs a minimum of 18–20 oz. of breast or formula milk a day, inclusive of milk used for mixing food. Babies who start to be weaned at six months could still be having 4–6 milk feedings a day, which you need to reduce rapidly if solids are not to be refused.

Some babies who are still drinking large amounts of milk at six months may be resistant to the introduction of solids. If you find that your baby is fussy about taking solids, you should offer him only half his milk at the 11 a.m. feeding to encourage interest in the solid food. You should aim to have your baby on two meals a day within a couple of weeks of beginning solids. By the time he reaches seven months, regardless of when he began weaning, all babies should be well established on two meals a day, progressing to three meals consisting of a wide variety of foods from the different food groups.

A very hungry baby who is taking three full milk feedings a day, plus three solid meals, including protein, may need a small drink and a piece of fruit midmorning and afternoon.

At the end of six months, a typical day's menu may look something like this:

7–7:30 a.m.	**Breakfast**
	Breast-feed or 6–8 oz. of formula
	Oat cereal mixed with milk and fruit *or* toast with fruit spread
11:30 a.m.	**Lunch**
	Chicken, vegetable or lentil casserole *or* steamed fish with creamed vegetables
2:30 p.m.	**Midafternoon**
	Breast-feed or 5–7 oz. of formula
5 p.m.	**Tea**
	Baked potato with vegetables *or* pasta with tomato sauce. Custard *or* yogurt. Small drink of water from a cup
6:30 p.m.	Breast-feed or 6–8 oz. of formula

Once a baby is established on three solid meals a day, plus 3–4 full milk feedings, he should manage to go close to 12 hours without a feeding. If your baby is not cutting down on his late feeding once solids are introduced, it may be that he is not getting the right quantities of solids for his age or weight or too small a feeding at 6:30 p.m. Keep a diary of all food and milk consumed over a period of four days to help pinpoint why he is not cutting that last feeding.

By the end of six months, your baby will probably be ready to sit in a high chair for his meals. Always ensure that he is properly strapped in and never left unattended.

. . . .

Second Stage: 7–9 Months

During the second stage of weaning, the amount of milk your baby drinks will gradually reduce as his intake of solids increases. It is, however, important that he still receives a minimum of 18–20 oz. a day of breast milk or formula. This is usually divided between three milk feedings and milk used in food and cooking, as sauces are introduced. At this stage of weaning you should be aiming at establishing three solid meals a day, so that by the time your baby reaches nine months of age he is getting most of his nourishment from solids. During this time, it is important to keep introducing a wide variety of food from the different food groups (carbohydrate, protein, dairy, fruit and vegetables) so that your baby's nutritional needs are met.

Most babies are ready to accept stronger-tasting food at this age. They also take pleasure from different textures, colors and presentation. Food should be mashed or "pulsed" and kept separate on the plate to avoid mixing everything up. Fruit need not be cooked; it can be grated or mashed. It is also around this age that your baby will begin to feed himself. Raw soft fruit, lightly cooked vegetables and toast can be used as finger food. They will be sucked and squeezed more than eaten at this stage, but allowing your baby the opportunity to feed himself encourages good eating habits later on. Once your baby is having finger food, always wash his hands before a meal and *never* leave him alone while he is eating.

During the second stage of weaning, when your baby increases the types of food that he eats, you can start to plan

. . . . . .

meals that are suitable for all the family. When giving your baby casseroles, you will still have to puree or pulse the meat: simply remove a portion of the meat, along with a little of the liquid, and puree or pulse to a texture that your baby will accept. Then serve with the appropriate amount of vegetables in the casserole. At this stage you may still have to chop or slice the vegetables smaller, but it is important that you start to move away from serving whole meals pulsed or pureed.

Between eight and nine months your baby may show signs of wanting to use his spoon. To encourage this, use two spoons when you feed him. Load one for him to try to get the food into his mouth. Use the other for actually getting the food in! You can help your baby's coordination by holding his wrist gently and guiding the spoon into his mouth. Finger food should also be offered at every meal at this stage.

Food to Introduce

Dairy products, pasta and wheat can be introduced at this stage. Full-fat cow's milk can be used in cooking but should not be given as a drink until the baby is one year old. Small amounts of unsalted butter can also be used in cooking. Egg yolk can be introduced, but it must be hardboiled. Cheese should be full fat, pasteurized, grated, and preferably organic. Olive oil can be used when cooking casseroles.

Canned fish such as tuna may also be included, but choose cans with a low-salt content. A greater variety of vegetables can also be introduced, such as colored peppers, brussels sprouts, pumpkin, cabbage and spinach.

Tomatoes and well-diluted unsweetened fruit juices can be included if your baby has no history of allergies. All these foods should be introduced gradually and careful notes made of any reactions.

Once your baby is used to taking food from a spoon, vegetables can be mashed rather than pureed. Once he is happy taking mashed food, you can start to introduce small amounts of finger food. Vegetables should be cooked until soft then offered in cube-sized pieces or steamed and then mixed to the right consistency.

When your baby is managing to feed himself softly cooked pieces of vegetables and soft pieces of raw fruit, you can try him with toast or a low-sugar cookie. By nine months, if your baby has several teeth, he should be able to manage some chopped raw vegetables. Dried fruit can also be given now, but it should be washed first.

Breakfast

Low-sugar, unrefined wheat cereals can now be introduced; choose those fortified with iron and B vitamins. You may want to delay introducing these if you have a family history of allergies—check with your pediatrician. Try adding a little mashed or grated fruit if your baby refuses them. Alternate the cereals between oat-based and wheat-based, even if your baby shows a preference for one over the other. You can encourage your baby with finger foods by offering him a little buttered toast. Once your baby is finger feeding, you can also offer a selection of fruits and yogurts.

Some babies are still desperate for their milk first thing in the morning, and if your baby still is, allow him two-thirds of his milk first. Once he is close to nine months of age, he will most likely show signs of not being hungry for milk, and this is the time to try offering breakfast milk from a cup.

Lunch

If your baby is eating a proper breakfast, you will be able to push lunch to somewhere between 11:45 a.m. and noon. However, should he be eating only a small amount of breakfast, lunch will need to come slightly earlier. Likewise, babies who are having only a very short nap in the morning may also need to have lunch earlier. It's important to remember that overtired, hungry babies will not eat well, so take your timing of lunch from your baby.

By this stage of weaning, you will have established protein at lunchtime. Whenever possible, buy organic meat as it is free from additives and growth hormones. Pork, bacon and processed hams should not be introduced until 18 months as they have a high-salt content. You should still continue to cook without additional salt or sugar, although a small amount of herbs can be introduced at around nine months of age.

If you are introducing your baby to a vegetarian diet, it is important to seek expert advice on getting the right balance of amino acids. Vegetables are incomplete sources of amino acids when cooked separately and need to be combined correctly to provide your baby with a complete source of protein.

Once protein is well established, replace your baby's milk at lunchtime with a drink of cool, boiled water or well-diluted juice from a cup. You might find that he only drinks a small amount from the cup and looks for an increase of milk on the 2:30 p.m. feeding or an increase of cool, boiled water later in the day.

If your baby is still hungry after his main meal, offer a piece of cheese, a breadstick, chopped fruit or yogurt.

Late-afternoon Snack

Once your baby is finger feeding, the late-afternoon snack can include a selection of mini-sandwiches. Baked potatoes or pasta served with vegetables and sauces are also suitable, although he will need help eating these. Some babies get very tired and fussy by this time of day. If your baby does not eat much, try offering some rice pudding or cereal. A small drink of water from a cup can be offered after the food. Do not allow too large a drink at this time as it will throw off his bedtime milk feeding, which is still important at this stage. If he starts cutting back too much on this feeding, check you are not overfeeding him on solids or giving him too much to drink.

Daily Requirements

At this second stage of weaning, it is important that you work toward establishing your baby on three proper meals a day. They should include three servings of carbohydrates, such as cereals, bread and pasta, at least three servings of vegetables and fruit and one serving of pureed meat, fish or beans. As his requirements of iron between six and twelve months are particularly high, it is important that his diet provides the right amount of iron. To help absorption of iron in cereals and meat, always serve them with fruit or vegetables and avoid giving milk to drink with protein as it reduces the iron content by 50 percent.

Your baby still needs 18–20 oz. of breast milk or formula a day, inclusive of milk used for mixing food. If your baby starts to reject his milk, try reducing the amount of solids you give him at the late-afternoon snack. By the end of nine months, encourage your baby to drink all of his breakfast milk from a cup. Apart from his bedtime milk, all drinks should be from a cup.

A very hungry baby who is taking three full milk feedings a day, plus three solid meals, may need a small drink and a piece of fruit midmorning.

A typical day's menu for an 8–9-month-old baby would look like this:

7–7:30 a.m.	**Breakfast** Breast-feed or 7–8 oz. of formula milk in a cup Mixed mashed fruit and yogurt *or* wheat/oat cereal with milk and mashed fruit
11:45 a.m./ noon	**Lunch** Chicken, broccoli and pasta in sauce *or* fish cakes with zucchini and potatoes; fruit and yogurt Drink of water or well-diluted juice from a cup
2:30 p.m.	**Midafternoon** Breast-feed or 5–6 oz. of formula milk in a cup
5 p.m.	**Late-afternoon snack** Baked potato with grated cheese and apple *or* vegetable lasagna Drink of water or well-diluted juice from a cup
6:30 p.m.	Breast-feed or 6–8 oz. of formula milk

Third Stage: 9–12 Months

Between 9 and 12 months your baby should be eating and enjoying all types of food, with the exception of food with a high-fat, -salt or -sugar content. Peanuts and honey should still be avoided. It is very important that your baby learns to chew properly at this stage. Food should be chopped or diced, although meat still needs to be pulsed or very finely chopped. By the end of his first year, your baby should be able to manage chopped meat. This is also a good time to introduce raw vegetables and salads. Include some finger foods at every meal, and if he shows an interest in holding his own spoon, do not discourage these attempts. When he repeatedly puts it into his mouth, load up his spoon and let him try to get it into his mouth, quickly popping in any food that falls out with your spoon. With a little help and guidance, starting at 12 months most babies are capable of feeding themselves part of their meal. It is important that he enjoys his meals even if a certain amount of it lands on the floor.

Breakfast

Aim to get your baby to have 7 oz. of milk at this meal, divided between a drink and his breakfast cereal. Scrambled egg can be offered once or twice a week as a change.

Ensure that you still offer milk at the start of the meal. Once he has taken 5–6 oz. of his milk, offer him some cereal. Then offer him the remainder of his milk again. It is important that he has at least 6–8 oz. of milk divided between the cup and the breakfast cereal. If you are still breast-feeding, offer him the first breast, then the solids and then offer him the breast again.

Between 9 and 12 months, a baby needs a minimum of 18 oz. of milk a day (inclusive of milk used in cooking or on cereal) divided between two or three milk feedings. This total also includes yogurt and cheese. As a guide, a 4-oz. serving of yogurt or a 1-oz. piece of cheese is the equivalent of approximately 7 oz. of milk.

Lunch

Lunch should consist of a wide selection of lightly steamed chopped vegetables and a serving of carbohydrates in the form of potato, pasta or rice served with a serving of protein. Babies of this age are very active and can become quite tired and irritable by 5 p.m. By ensuring a well-balanced lunch, you will not need to worry if the late-afternoon snack is more relaxed. By the end of the first year, your baby's lunch can be integrated with the family meal. Prepare the food without salt, sugar or spices, reserve a portion for your baby and then add the desired flavorings for the rest of the family.

Try to ensure that his meals are attractively presented, with a variety of different-colored vegetables and fruit. Do not overload his plate; serve up a small amount and, when he finishes that, replenish his plate. This also helps to avoid the game of throwing food on the floor, which often occurs at this stage. If your baby does start to play with his main course, refusing to eat and throwing food around, quietly and firmly say no and remove the plate. Do *not* offer him a cookie or yogurt half an hour later, as a pattern will soon emerge in which he will refuse lunch knowing he will get something sweet if he plays enough. A piece of fruit can be offered midafternoon to see him through to his late-afternoon snack, at which time he will probably eat very well.

A drink of well-diluted pure, unsweetened orange juice in a cup will help the absorption of iron at this meal, but make sure your baby has most of his meal before you allow him to finish the drink.

The 2:30 P.M. Feeding

By 9–12 months, bottle-fed babies should be given most of their milk from a cup, which should automatically result in a decrease in the amount they drink. If your baby starts to cut back on his last milk feeding, reduce, or cut out altogether, the 2:30 p.m. feeding. Many babies cut out the 2:30 p.m. feeding by one year. At 12 months, as long as your baby is getting a minimum of 12 oz. of milk a day, inclusive of milk used in cereal and cooking, he will be getting enough. If he is getting 18 oz. of milk a day (inclusive of milk used in cooking, on cereal and in cheese and yogurt), plus a full, balanced diet of solids, you could cut this feeding altogether.

Once your baby has dropped this feeding, it can be replaced by a small snack (for example a rice cake, an unsweetened cookie or a small piece of fruit) and a drink of water or very well-diluted juice from a cup.

Late-afternoon Snack

Many babies cut out their 2:30 p.m. milk during this stage. If you are worried that your baby's daily milk intake is too low, try giving him things like pasta and vegetables with a milk sauce, baked potatoes with grated cheese, cheesy vegetable bake or mini-quiches at the late-afternoon snack. This is usually the meal when I would give small helpings of custard or yogurt, which are also alternatives if milk is being rejected. Try regularly to include some finger foods at the 5 p.m. snack time.

The bedtime bottle should be discouraged after one year, so during this stage get your baby gradually used to less milk at bedtime. This can be done by offering him a small drink of milk with his late-afternoon snack, then a drink of 5–6 oz. of milk from a cup at bedtime.

The 6–7 P.M. Feeding

By 10–12 months, bottle-fed babies should be taking all of their milk from a cup. Babies who continue to feed from a bottle after one year are more prone to feeding problems, as they continue to take large amounts of milk, which takes the edge off their appetite for solids.

Start encouraging your baby to take some of his milk from a cup at nine months, so that by one year he is happy to give up his bottles.

Daily Requirements

By one year, it is important that large volumes of milk are discouraged; no more than 20 oz., inclusive of milk used in food, should be allowed. More than this can adversely affect his appetite for solid food. After one year, your baby needs a minimum of 12 oz. a day. This is usually divided between two or three drinks and is inclusive of milk used in cooking or on cereals.

Full-fat, pasteurized cow's milk can be given to drink after one year. If your baby refuses this, try gradually diluting his formula with it until it is completely switched over. If possible, give your baby grass-fed cow's milk as it has more Omega 3 essential fatty acids than nonorganic milk. Omega 3 fatty acids are essential for maintaining a healthy heart, supple and flexible joints, healthy growth and strong bones and teeth so it is important to make sure your baby is getting enough of them through his food. All bottles or cups used for formula milk should be sterilized until your baby is 12 months old.

Aim to give your baby three well-balanced meals a day and avoid snacks of cookies, cakes and crackers. Every day, aim for him to have 3–4 servings of carbohydrate, 3–4 servings of fruit and vegetables, and one portion of animal protein or two of vegetable protein.

By one year, your baby's menu should look something like this:

7–7:30 a.m.	**Breakfast**
	Breast-feed or a drink of formula in a cup
	Whole wheat or oat cereal with milk and fruit *or* baby muesli with milk and fruit *or* scrambled egg on toast *or* yogurt and chopped fruit
Noon	**Lunch**
	Chicken with apple and cucumbers *or* meatballs in tomato sauce with roasted potatoes *or* tuna burgers and mixed vegetables
	Drink of water or well-diluted juice from a cup
	Yogurt and fresh fruit
2:30 p.m.	**Midafternoon**
	Drink of milk, water or well-diluted juice from a cup
5 p.m.	**Late-afternoon snack**
	Thick soup with a sandwich *or* vegetarian pizza with green salad *or* chickpea and spinach croquettes with sauce *or* lentil and vegetable lasagna
	Small drink of milk, water or well-diluted juice from a cup
6:30 p.m.	Breast-feed or 6 oz. of formula milk from a cup

Your Questions Answered

Q How will I know when my baby is ready to be weaned?

A Your baby has been sleeping through and starts to wake in the night or very early in the morning, and will not settle back to sleep.

* A bottle-fed baby would be taking in excess of 32–38 oz. a day, draining an 8-oz. bottle each feeding and looking for another feeding long before it is due.

* A breast-fed baby would start to look for a feeding every 2–3 hours.

* Both breast- and bottle-fed babies would start to chew on their hands a lot and be very irritable in between feedings.

✳ If unsure, talk to your pediatrician, especially if your baby is less than six months old.

Q What would happen if I weaned my baby before he was ready?

A His digestive system could be harmed if he has not developed the complete set of enzymes required to digest solids.

✳ Introducing solids before he is ready could lead to allergies.

✳ Studies from several different countries show that persistent coughs and wheezing are more common in babies that were weaned before 17 weeks.

Q At what milk feeding should I introduce solids?

A I usually start at the 11 a.m. feeding as this one will gradually be pushed to noon, becoming a proper lunch once solids become established by the end of the first year.

✳ Milk is still the most important source of food. By giving solids after this feeding, you can be sure that your baby will have at least half of his daily milk intake before noon.

✳ Solids offered at the 2:30 p.m. feeding seem to put babies off the very important 6 p.m. feeding.

✳ If a very hungry baby has no adverse reaction to the baby rice within three days, I would then transfer the rice to after the 6 p.m. feeding.

Q **Which is the best food to introduce?**

A I find pure organic baby rice is the food that satisfies most babies' hunger the best. If this is tolerated I would then introduce some organic pureed pear.

＊ Once these two foods are established, it is best to concentrate on introducing a variety of vegetables from the How to Begin stage earlier in this chapter.

Q **How will I know how much solid food to give my baby?**

A For the first six months, milk is still the most important part of your baby's diet. It will provide him with the right balance of vitamins and minerals, so once solids are introduced, he will need a minimum of 20 oz. a day. During the first weeks of weaning, if you always offer the milk feeding first, then the solids, you can be sure he will take exactly the amount of solids he needs. This avoids him replacing his milk too quickly with solids.

＊ Once you have established rice and some purees, you can start at the 11 a.m. feeding to give half the milk feeding first, then some solids followed by more milk. This will encourage your baby to cut back slightly on his milk feeding and increase his solids, preparing him for an eating pattern of three meals a day at seven months.

＊ For breast-fed babies, a feeding from one breast can be classed as half a milk feeding.

Q **At what age do I start to cut out milk feedings altogether?**

A Assuming your baby was on five milk feedings when he started to wean, once he increases his solids after the 6 p.m. feeding, he should automatically cut back on his late feeding, then cut it out altogether. If you wean at six months, you will probably need to keep the late feeding. Once solids are established it should be easy to cut it out.

* The next feeding to cut out would be the 11–11:30 a.m. feeding. Once your baby is having chicken or fish for lunch the milk feeding should be replaced with a drink of water or well-diluted juice from a cup.

* The 2:30 p.m. feeding often increases for a few months then, somewhere between 9 and 12 months, he will lose interest in this feeding, at which time it can be dropped.

Q **At what age would you introduce a drinking cup and at which feedings?**

A The best time is between six and seven months.

* When you have replaced the lunchtime milk feeding with water or well-diluted juice, try giving it from a cup or a sippy cup.

* Try halfway through the meal and after every few spoonfuls of food.

* It is important to persevere. Experiment with different types of cups until you find one with which your baby is happy.

✳ Once he is taking a few ounces from a cup, gradually introduce it at other feedings.

Q **When can I introduce cow's milk?**

A I usually introduce a small amount of organic cow's milk in cooking from six months.

✳ Cow's milk should not be given as a drink until your baby is at least one year old.

✳ It should always be full-fat, pasteurized milk, preferably organic.

✳ If your baby refuses cow's milk, try mixing half that amount with formula. Once he is happy taking that, gradually increase the cow's milk until he is happy with all cow's milk.

Q **At what age can I stop pureeing my baby's food?**

A Once your baby has taken well to pureed food (hopefully by the end of the sixth month), you can start to mash the vegetables and fruit really well, so that there are no lumps, but it is not as smooth as the pureed food.

✳ Between six and nine months, I gradually mash the food less and less until the babies will take food with lumps in it.

✳ Chicken and meat should still be pureed until your baby is around 10 months old.

Q When will he be able to spoon-feed himself?

A Once your baby starts to grab at the spoon, give him one to hold.

* When he repeatedly puts it in his mouth, load up the spoon and let him try to get it into his mouth, quickly popping in with your spoon any food that falls out.

* With a little help and guidance, most babies 12 months and older are capable of feeding themselves part of their meal.

* Always supervise your baby during mealtimes. Never, ever leave him alone.

Q When can I stop sterilizing?

A Bottles should be sterilized until your baby is one year old.

* You can stop sterilizing dishes and spoons when your baby is six months old. They can then be put into the dishwasher or washed thoroughly in hot soapy water, then rinsed and left to air-dry.

* After six months, the pots, cooking utensils and ice cube trays used for preparing weaning food can either be put into the dishwasher or washed in hot soapy water, rinsed and doused with boiled water poured over them before being left to air-dry. If you are weaning before six months, the equipment should be sterilized.

Q Which foods are most likely to cause allergies, and what are the main symptoms?

A The foods that most often cause allergies are dairy products, wheat, fish, eggs and citrus fruits.

* Symptoms include rashes, wheezing, coughing, running nose, sore bottom, diarrhea, irritability and swelling of the eyes.

* Keeping a detailed record when you are weaning can be a big help when you are trying to establish the cause of any of these symptoms.

* House mites, animal fur, wool and certain soaps and household cleaning agents can also cause these symptoms.

* If in doubt, always check with your doctor to rule out any other possible causes for the above symptoms.

16

Problem Solving in the First Year

• • • • • •

The advice in this book is based on the hundreds of babies I have personally cared for. Each baby is an individual, and it is natural that problems may occur. Drawing on the feedback from my Web site and consultancy service, I have focused on the most common problems encountered by parents during the first year, and this chapter should cover the majority of your concerns. Remember to consult your pediatrician with any worries—even if they seem small and you fear looking like a neurotic mother. It's better that you are not beset with worries and can enjoy your baby and this precious first year together.

I have divided the information in this chapter into three sections—general, feeding and sleeping problems—but many of them overlap. Sleeping and feeding are interdependent, so you may find it more helpful to read both of those sections.

. . . .

General Problems

Burping

It is important to follow your baby's lead regarding when to stop and burp him during feeding. If you constantly interrupt his meal trying to burp him, he will more likely get so upset and frustrated that the crying will cause more wind than the feeding itself. Time and time again, I watch babies being thumped endlessly on the back, the mother refusing to continue with the feeding as she is convinced the baby has gas. The reality is that very few babies need to be burped more than once during a feeding and once at the end.

A breast-fed baby will pull himself off the breast when he is ready to burp. If he has not done so by the end of the first breast, you can try burping him before putting him on the second breast. Bottle-fed babies will normally drink half to three-quarters of their bottle and pull themselves off to be burped. Regardless of whether you are breast-feeding or bottle-feeding, if you adopt the correct holding position as illustrated in Chapter Three, Milk Feeding in the First Year, your baby should bring his gas up quickly and easily both during and at the end of the feeding. If your baby does not bring up the wind within a few minutes, it is best to try again later. More often than not, he will bring it up after he has been laid flat for his diaper change.

Occasionally, a baby passing excessive gas from his rear end can suffer considerable discomfort and become very distressed. A breast-feeding mother should keep a close eye on her diet to see if a particular food or drink is causing the gas. Citrus fruits or drinks taken in excess by the mother can sometimes cause

. . . . . .

severe gas in babies. The other culprits are chocolate and excessive dairy intake.

Special care should be taken to make sure that the baby is reaching the hind milk. Too much fore milk can cause explosive bowel movements and excessive passing of gas.

With a bottle-fed baby who is already feeding from special anticolic bottles, the cause of excessive gas is usually overfeeding. If your baby is regularly drinking 3–6 oz. a day more than the amount advised on the packet and constantly putting on in excess of 8 oz. of weight each week, cut back on a couple of his feedings (either the 2:30 p.m. or 5 p.m.) for a few days to see if there is any improvement. A "sucky" baby could be offered a pacifier after the smaller feedings to satisfy his sucking needs.

Sometimes a nipple with a hole either too small or too large for your baby's needs can cause excessive gas. Experiment with the different sizes of nipples; sometimes using a smaller hole at a couple of the feedings can help a baby who is drinking some of his feedings too quickly.

Colic

Colic is a common problem for babies less than three months. It can make life miserable for the baby and the parents, and to date, there is no cure for it. There are over-the-counter medications, but most parents with a baby suffering from severe colic say that they are of little help. Although a baby can suffer from colic at any time of the day, the most common time seems to be between 6 p.m. and midnight. Parents resort to endless feeding, rocking, patting, driving the baby around the block, most of which seem to bring little or no relief. Colic usually disappears by four months of age; but by that time, the baby has often learned all the wrong sleep associations, so the parents are no further ahead.

Parents who contact me for help with their colicky baby describe how the baby screams, often for hours at a time, thrashes madly and keeps bringing his legs up in pain. These babies seem to have one thing in common: They are all being fed on demand. Feeding this way all too often leads to the baby having a feeding before the first one has been digested, one of the causes, I believe, of colic.

Not one of the babies I have cared for has ever suffered from colic, and I am convinced that it is because I structure their feeding and sleeping from day one. When I do go in to help an older baby who is suffering from colic, it seems to disappear within 24 hours of him being put on the routine.

First, I would check that colic was being caused by demand-feeding and not the mother's diet. Then, depending upon the age of the baby, the symptoms, and how often he was feeding throughout the evening and the middle of the night, I would introduce sugar water. With a baby between one and three months of age who was feeding excessively in the night and consistently putting on more than the recommended weight gain each week, I would replace one of the night feedings with some sugar water. When the baby woke in the night, I would give 2 oz. of cool boiled water mixed with half a teaspoon of sugar to settle him. At this stage, I find plain boiled water does not have the same effect. The following day I would wake the baby at 7 a.m., regardless of how little sleep he had in the night, and then proceed with the routine throughout the day until 6:30 p.m. At this time, I would always offer a breast-fed baby a top-up of expressed milk to ensure that he has had enough to drink. This avoids his need to feed again in two hours, which is a common pattern of babies suffering from colic. With a bottle-fed baby I always make sure that the 2:30 p.m. feeding is smaller so that he eats well at 6:30 p.m.

......

With a baby of three months or more, I would attempt to eliminate middle-of-the-night feedings altogether or at least reduce the feeding to only one. In both cases, it is important to ensure that the baby eats well at 6:15 p.m., if necessary by offering a top-up of expressed milk at this time. A low milk supply in the early evening is often the cause of a baby feeding little and often, which can lead to him not digesting properly.

More often than not, the baby settles well the first night, but occasionally I worked with a baby who had developed the wrong sleep associations as a result of colic. With these babies I used the crying-down method of sleep training and within 3–4 nights they were going down happily and sleeping well until the late feeding. Because they had slept well and had gone a full four hours since their last feeding, they fed well and went on to last for an even longer spell in the night. Depending upon their age, they were given either a feeding or sugar water. A baby of three months or older who is capable of going from the last feeding through to 6–7 a.m. should be given sugar water for a week. Once the pattern of once-a-night waking is established, gradually reduce the amount of sugar until he is taking plain water.

This method, along with the routines, will encourage a baby who has suffered from colic and developed the wrong sleep associations to sleep through the night, normally within a couple of weeks. I cannot stress strongly enough that the success of this method very much depends upon the use of the sugar water during the first week. Plain water does not have the same success. I picked up this tip from an older maternity nurse more than 25 years ago, and it has never failed me. Parents are often concerned that it will encourage their babies to develop a sweet tooth, or even worse, rot their teeth. Because of the short period the sugar water is used, I have never seen any of these problems evolve. I am also pleased to say that my advice has now been backed up by recent research on colic by Dr. Peter Lewindon of the Royal Children's Hospital, Brisbane, Australia. Research shows that sugar stimulates the body's natural painkillers and that some babies suffering from colic can be helped by the sugar water solution.

Crying

According to the American Academy of Pediatrics, newborns routinely cry a total of 1–4 hours a day. With very young babies, I have noticed that they do go through unsettled stages around 3–6 weeks, which tends to coincide with growth spurts. However, I would be absolutely horrified if any of my babies cried for even one hour a day, let alone 2–4 hours! The one thing that parents comment upon time and time again is how happy their baby is on the routine. Of course, my babies do cry; some when they have their diaper changed, others when having their face washed, and a few when fighting sleep when put in their crib. With the ones that fight sleep, because I know that they are well fed, burped and ready to sleep, I am very strict. I let them fuss and yell for 10–12 minutes until they have settled themselves. This is the only real crying I experience, and even then, it occurs with the minority of my babies and lasts for no longer than a week or two. Understandably, all parents hate to hear their baby cry; many are worried that to put their baby in a crib to sleep and leave him to cry like this could be psychologically damaging. I would like to reassure you that, provided your baby has been well fed, and you have followed the routines regarding awake periods and winding-down time, your baby will not suffer psychological damage. In the long term, you will have a happy, contented baby who has learned to settle himself to sleep. Many parents who have followed the demand method with the first baby, and my routines with their second baby, would confirm wholeheartedly that my methods are by far better and, in the long term, easier.

Marc Weissbluth, M.D., Director of the Sleep Disorders Center at the Children's Memorial Hospital, Chicago, says in his book, *Healthy Sleep Habits, Happy Child* that parents should remember they are *allowing* their baby to cry, not *making* him cry. He also says that it will be much harder for an older baby to learn how to settle himself. Therefore, do not feel guilty or cruel if you have to allow a short spell of crying when your baby is going to sleep. He will very quickly learn to settle himself as long as you have made sure he is well fed and has been awake long enough but not so long that he has become overtired.

Following are the main reasons a healthy baby would cry. Use them as a checklist. At the top of that list is hunger. A tiny baby who is hungry should always be fed, regardless of routines.

Hunger

When your baby is very tiny and fretful and unsettled, it is, of course, wise to assume that when he cries the problem is hunger and to offer him milk or formula, even if it is before the time recommended in the routine for his age. One of the main reasons that I find very young breast-fed babies are unsettled in the evening is usually hunger. If your baby eats well, stays awake for a short spell after feedings, then sleeps well until the next feeding but is unsettled in the evening—it is very possible the cause is hunger. Even if your baby is putting on a good amount of weight each week, you should not rule out hunger. Many mothers I know can produce a lot of milk early on in the day, but come the evening, when tiredness has crept in, the milk supply can decrease dramatically. I would strongly recommend that, for a few nights, you try topping him up with a small amount of expressed milk after his bath. If he settles well then you will know that your milk supply is low at that time of the evening. Please check "Low Milk Supply" later in this chapter for suggestions on how to deal with this problem.

However, if you find that your baby is unsettled in the evening, or indeed any other time of the day, despite being well fed, it is important that you eliminate other reasons for his fretfulness. During my many years of caring for young babies, I did have a handful who were very fretful in the early days, no matter what I did to help calm them. If I had a very unsettled baby I would go through every possibility before accepting that there was nothing I could do to help. Babies do have many needs other than feeding, sleeping and being held.

Tiredness

Babies less than six weeks tend to get tired after one hour of being awake. Although they may not be quite ready to sleep, they need to be kept quiet and calm. Not all babies show obvious signs of tiredness, so in the early days, after your baby has been awake for one hour, I still advise that you take him to his room, so he can wind down gradually. If you can't do that, at least try to keep him in a peaceful part of the house. Try not to allow visitors to overstimulate a baby during this winding-down period.

Overtiredness

No baby less than three months should be allowed to stay awake for more than two hours at a time, as he can become very overtired and difficult to settle.

Overtiredness is often a result of overstimulation. An overtired baby reaches a stage at which he is unable to drift off to sleep naturally, and the more tired he becomes, the more he fights sleep. A baby younger than three months who is allowed to get into this state and stays awake for more than two hours can become almost impossible to settle.

In a situation like this sometimes a short period of crying down has to be used as a last resort to solve the problem. This is the only situation when I would advise that young babies should be left to cry for a short period, and even then, it can only be done if you are confident that the baby has been well fed and burped.

Boredom

Even a newborn baby needs to be awake some of the time. Encourage him to be awake for a short spell after his day feedings. Babies less than one month love to look at anything black and white, especially pictures of faces, and the ones that fascinate them most will be the faces of their parents. Divide the toys into ones that are used for wakeful periods and ones that are used for winding-down time. Bright, noisy ones for social time; calm, soothing ones for sleepy times.

Gas

All babies pass a certain amount of gas while feeding, bottle-fed babies more so than breast-fed ones. Given the opportunity, most babies bring up their gas easily. If you suspect that your baby's crying is caused by gas, check that you are allowing enough time between feedings. I have found overfeeding and demand-feeding to be the main causes of colic in young babies.

A breast-fed baby needs at least three hours to digest a full feeding, and a formula-fed baby should be allowed 3½–4 hours. This time is always from the beginning of one feeding to the beginning of the next one.

I would also suggest that you keep a close eye on your baby's weight gain. If his weight gain exceeds 8–10 oz. a week and he appears to be suffering from gas pains, it could be that he is overfeeding, particularly if he weighs more than 8 lbs. and is feeding 2–3 times in the night. For details on how to deal with this problem refer to Chapter Three, Milk Feeding in the First Year.

Pacifiers

I have always believed that, if used with discretion, a pacifier can be a great asset, especially for a sucky baby. The Mayo Clinic reports on its Web site that to reduce the risk of SIDS, the American Academy of Pediatrics recommends offering a pacifier at nap time or bedtime until age one. However, I have always stressed the importance of never allowing the baby to have the pacifier in his crib or of allowing him to suck himself to sleep on the pacifier. My advice was that it is fine to use it to calm a baby and, if necessary, settle him at sleep times, but it must be removed before he falls asleep. In my experience, allowing a baby to fall asleep with a pacifier in his mouth is one of the worst sleep-association problems to solve. He can end up waking several times a night, and each time he will expect the pacifier to get back to sleep.

There are two types of pacifiers available: one has a round cherry-type nipple; the other has a flat-shaped nipple, which is called an orthodontic nipple. Some experts claim that the orthodontic nipple shape is better for the baby's mouth, but the problem with this type is that most young babies cannot hold them in for very long. I tend to use the cherry-type nipple, and so far, none of my babies appears to have developed an overbite, which is often the result of a pacifier being used excessively once the teeth have come through. Whichever type of pacifier you choose, buy several so that they can be changed frequently. The utmost attention should be paid to cleanliness when using a pacifier; it should be washed and sterilized after each use. Never clean it by licking it, as so many parents do; there are more germs and bacteria in the mouth than you would believe.

Hiccups

Hiccups are very normal among tiny babies, and very few become distressed by them. Hiccups often happen after a feeding. If it has been a nighttime feeding and your baby is due to go down for a sleep, it is advisable to go ahead and put him down regardless. If you wait until the hiccups are finished, there is a bigger chance of him falling asleep in your arms, which is something to be avoided at all costs. If your baby is one of the rare ones who gets upset by hiccups, then try giving him the recommended dose of gripe water, which can sometimes help.

Spitting Up

It is very common for babies to bring up a small amount of milk while being burped or after a feeding. It is called spitting up, and for most babies it does not create a problem. However, if your baby is regularly gaining more than 8 oz. of weight each week, spitting up could be a sign that he is drinking too much. With a bottle-fed baby, the problem is easily solved as you are able to see how much the baby is drinking and, therefore, slightly reduce the amount at the feedings during which he appears to spit up more. It is more difficult to tell how much a breast-fed baby is drinking. But by keeping a note of which feedings cause more spitting up and reducing the time on the breast at those feedings, the spitting up may be reduced.

If your baby is spitting up excessively and not gaining weight it could be that he is suffering from a condition called reflux (see the next section). With babies who are inclined to bring up milk, it is important to keep them as upright as possible after a feeding and special care should be taken when burping.

Any baby bringing up an entire feeding twice in a row should be seen by a doctor immediately.

Reflux

Sometimes a baby displaying all the symptoms of colic actually has a condition called gastroesophageal reflux. Because the muscle at the lower end of the esophagus is too weak to keep the milk in the baby's stomach, it comes back up, along with acid from the stomach, causing a very painful burning sensation in the esophagus. Excessive spitting up is one of the symptoms of reflux. However, not all babies with reflux actually spit up the milk; some suffer from what the medical profession calls silent reflux. These babies are often misdiagnosed as having colic. They can be very difficult to feed, constantly arching their backs and screaming during a feeding. They also tend to become very irritable when laid flat, and no amount of cuddling or rocking will calm them when they are like this. If your baby displays these symptoms, insist that your doctor does a reflux test. I have seen too many cases of babies being diagnosed as having colic, when in fact they were suffering from reflux. If you think that your baby is suffering from reflux, it is essential that you do not allow anyone to dismiss the pains as colic. Reflux is very stressful for the baby and parents, and it is essential that you get on-going advice and support from your doctor. If you feel that you are not getting the help you need, do not be afraid to ask for a second opinion. If reflux is not the problem, you will at least have eliminated it as a possible cause. If it is the problem, with the right medication your baby will have been saved months of misery. It is important that a baby with reflux is not overfed and is kept as upright as possible during and after feeding. Some babies may need medication for several months until the muscles of the esophagus tighten up. Fortunately, the majority of babies outgrow the condition by the time they are one year old.

If your baby is diagnosed with reflux, it is worth looking at the reflux section on my Web site www.contentedbaby.com. There you will find case studies, plus lots of advice and tips on how to survive those early months with a reflux baby.

Separation Anxiety

At about the age of six months, babies start to gain more understanding of their environment and begin to realize that they are separate from their mother. Between the ages of 6 and 12 months, most babies show some signs of separation anxiety. You may find that your happy, contented baby, who was so easygoing and relaxed, suddenly becomes clingy, anxious and demanding, and starts crying the minute you leave the room.

This sudden change of your baby's temperament can be very upsetting, but do be reassured that this behavior is a totally normal part of a baby's development. All babies go through this stage to some degree.

Although this stage can be a very exhausting time for you, it rarely lasts long. The following guidelines can help make this difficult period less stressful:

✳ A comforter can be very reassuring to babies and can provide a consistent comforting familiarity. Consider introducing one if your child hasn't already made an attachment. Often a baby will choose his own comforter, and these are generally a familiar object with comforting associations, such as a soft toy, a crib blanket or a burp cloth. If you choose to guide your baby, choose a toy that can be replaced (a spare cuddly toy that is interchanged regularly is a very sensible precaution). You should also think of the practicalities. Safety is paramount—you need to make sure that the comforter has no loose pieces that could prove a choking hazard. It should be washable and durable. It is extremely distressing for both your baby and you if the comforter is mislaid, so it might be worth encouraging your baby to leave the comforter at home on trips to the park or on play dates.

✳ Aim to get your baby used to whatever child care you have chosen. Ideally give both of you one month to become accustomed to the situation. Lengthen the time you leave the baby in stages.

✳ The longer you give yourself and your child the time to get used to a separation, the more flexibility you will have. For instance, if your baby is inconsolable by your departure, you might delay trying to leave him again for a week or so. With such a young child, every day adds to his confidence and understanding, and it might be that if you wait a week or so, your baby will have a different response next time you leave him.

✳ If your baby has a particular activity he enjoys—hitting a saucepan with a spoon or playing with a particular toy—have your baby's child-care provider have something similar to offer.

* Try role-playing. Even very young babies can grasp the concept of people or toys leaving and returning. Maybe encourage your baby to say "good-bye" to a doll or teddy bear, and then "hello."

* Praise your child when he is prepared to go with your child-care provider.

* Talk to your baby. It is extraordinary how much a little baby can take in. If your baby is used to his father leaving for work each day, keep repeating: "Daddy has gone to work." This will reinforce his confidence that when the time comes for Mommy to go to work, she will also be returning.

* When you prepare to leave your baby, make sure that you keep your good-bye to a minimum. Be positive, use reassuring phrases and smile; this will help to reassure him. Try a hug and kiss and a verbal reminder that you will be back soon. Using the same approach and words each time you say good-bye will, in the long term, be more reassuring than going back to calm him. While a baby will often cry when a parent leaves the room, most children will be easy to distract in the hands of a competent caregiver. However, babies are sensitive to moods, and if you are anxious and worried, your baby will pick up on this and be more likely to be upset.

* Avoid just slipping away when you leave your baby. Although you will find it difficult if he is upset when you say good-bye, it is much better for him to understand that you are going and that you will return rather than

for him to look around later to find that you have vanished. This could contribute to his unhappiness—he might become confused and clingy.

✳ Be realistic—you might well find that your baby is fretful at home even though the caregiver has told you that he is happy and content when you are not there. In the same way that you will find the change to your routine tiring, so will your baby. Don't worry; provided that the circumstances are loving and secure, babies are adaptable.

✳ During this period of adjustment, ask your baby's caregiver to ensure that your baby is not subjected to too many new experiences or handled by strangers. The calmer and more predictable his routine, the quicker he will get over his feelings of anxiety.

✳ If your baby is used to just being with you for the first six months, you can imagine that adapting to a livelier environment can be challenging. If you have chosen a child-care provider who also looks after other children, your baby will need to adapt to a noisier, more dynamic environment than he is used to. You can help your baby by arranging regular play dates with a small group of mothers and babies. Not only will this be enjoyable for you, but also it will enable your baby to get used to the noise and activity of other children. If you have a nervous baby, you will find that he will become happier once he is used to a different environment. Gradually introduce him to larger groups and other experiences. Generally babies love the activities of toddlers so, providing that they are appropriately monitored, you can feel reassured that it will be a pleasant experience for him.

Stranger Anxiety

At around six months, you might also find that your sociable baby is wary of strangers. This is a natural part of his development. It is thought that this fear of strangers is a biological protective response relating to our origins. It contributed to a baby's ability to survive in a primitive environment.

We have an expectation that babies are happy to be handed to loving relatives and friends for cuddles when they are small, but even small babies can find that being passed from one loving relative to the next is tiring and distressing.

* If your baby begins to cry when approached by strangers or to look away when someone is trying to engage him, don't attempt to push him to communicate. It is much better to explain that your child is becoming self-conscious and having a shy period than to expect your baby to smile on cue!
* You can ease this response to those friends and family you see regularly by talking to your baby about them. If you have a photo-montage on the wall, you can show your baby photographs and explain who they are.
* For those grandparents or family who see your baby more occasionally, it can be upsetting when your child is distressed or tearful but be reassured that any initial concern will not last long if you are in a position to spend some time together.
* Role-play can also help in this circumstance; try giving your baby's toys the names of the friends and family with whom you want him to be familiar.
* Consider asking friends to not make too much fuss over your baby upon first arriving. Sometimes a baby

can find their physical proximity threatening, and it is easier if the baby is allowed to respond in his own time, when he feels comfortable with the new person, rather than when someone is attempting to make eye contact and communicate.

✳ Although your baby will learn how to deal with greetings and attention as he grows up, some children remain shy. It is much better for you to adapt to this and try to understand how it feels to be a shy child, rather than pushing your child into situations in which he feels uncomfortable or distressed.

Common Feeding Problems

Difficult Feeder

The majority of newborn babies take to the breast or bottle quickly and easily. Unlike the new mother, who has much to learn about feeding, the baby instinctively knows what is expected of him. However, there are some babies who, from day one, will fuss and fret within minutes of being put on the breast or being offered the bottle. I often find that some babies who have undergone a particularly hard birth can be more difficult to feed.

If you find that your baby becomes tense and fretful at feeding times, try to avoid having visitors then. No matter how well-meaning family and friends may be, it will be impossible to keep things completely calm and quiet if you are having to make conversation. The following guidelines, regardless of whether you are breast- or bottle-feeding, should help make feeding a tense baby easier:

* It is essential that the handling of tense babies is kept to the minimum. Avoid overstimulation and handing the baby from person to person, especially before a feeding.
* Whenever possible, try to nurse in a quiet room with a calm atmosphere. Apart from perhaps one person to offer practical help and emotional support, no other person should be allowed in the room.
* Prepare everything needed for the feeding well in advance. Try to make sure that you have rested and eaten.
* Avoid turning on the television during a feeding; unplug the telephone and play some calm music while feeding.
* When the baby wakes for his feeding, do not change his diaper as this may trigger crying.
* Try swaddling him firmly in a soft receiving blanket to prevent him from thrashing his arms and legs around. Make sure that you are comfortable before you start feeding.
* Do not attempt to latch the baby onto the breast or put the bottle straight in his mouth if he is crying. Hold him firmly in the feeding position and calm him down with continuous gentle patting on the back.
* Try holding a pacifier in his mouth. Once he has calmed down and has sucked steadily for a few minutes, then very quickly ease the pacifier out and offer him the breast or the bottle.

If you find your baby is fussy when feeding and taking a lot longer than an hour to eat, try allowing him a short break halfway through the feeding. It is better to let your baby eat in two shorter spurts than spend a lengthy time trying to force him to eat.

If your baby has been eating well and suddenly starts to refuse the breast or bottle, it could be because he is feeling unwell. Ear infections can easily go undetected and are a very common cause of a baby not wanting to eat. If your baby shows any of the following signs it would be advisable to consult your doctor:

* Sudden loss of appetite, and becoming upset when offered a feeding.
* Disruption to the normal sleep pattern.
* Suddenly becoming clingy and whiney.
* Becoming lethargic and unsociable.

Low Milk Supply

As they grow, all babies will drink more. However, the feedings must be structured to coordinate with the baby's growth, thereby encouraging him to take more milk at each feeding. If not, he will be very likely to continue to feed little and often.

All too often, I get calls from the parents of older babies who are still following the demand rules of milk feeding. While the majority of these babies are more than 12 weeks old and are physically capable of drinking more at individual feedings, they continue to nurse as they did as newborns—often 8–10 times a day.

Many breast-fed babies are still having only one breast at each feeding, while bottle-fed babies may be taking only 3–4 oz. of formula. In order to go for longer spells between feedings, these babies should be taking from both breasts at each feeding, or have a formula feeding of 7–8 oz. It is my firm belief that it is during those early days of milk feeding that the foundation is laid for healthy eating habits in the future. To avoid long-term feeding problems that can affect your baby's sleep, it is advisable to structure and solve any milk-feeding problems early on.

Not producing enough milk, especially later in the day, is a very common problem for breast-feeding mothers and one of the major reasons breast-feeding goes wrong. I believe that hunger is why so many babies are fretful and difficult to settle in the evening. If the problem of a low milk supply is not re-solved in the early days, then a pattern soon emerges of the baby needing to feed on and off all evening to satisfy his needs. Mothers are advised that this constant feeding is normal and the best way to increase the milk supply, but in my experience, it usually has the opposite effect. Because the amount of milk the breasts produce is dictated by the amount of milk the baby drinks, these frequent feedings signal the breasts to produce milk little and often. These small feedings will rarely satisfy the baby, leaving him hungry and irritable.

I believe that the stress involved in frequently feeding a very hungry, irritable and often overtired baby can cause many mothers to become so exhausted that their milk supply is re-duced even further. Exhaustion and a low milk supply go hand in hand. I am convinced that by expressing a small amount of milk during the early weeks of breast-feeding, when the breasts are producing more milk than the baby needs, the mother can help avoid the problem of a low milk supply.

If your baby is less than one month of age and not settling in the evening, it is possible the cause is a low milk supply. Ex-pressing at the times I suggest should help solve this problem. The short amount of time you spend expressing will ensure that during any future growth spurts you will be producing enough milk to meet any increase in your baby's appetite. If your baby is more than one month and not settling in the evening or after daytime feedings, the following six-day plan will quickly help to increase your milk supply. The temporary introduction of top-up feedings will ensure that your baby is not subjected to hours of irritability and anxiety caused by hunger, which is what usually happens when mothers resort to demand feeding to increase their milk supply.

Plan for Increased Milk Supply

Days One to Three

6:45 A.M.
* Express 1 oz. from each breast.
* Baby should be awake, and eating no later than 7 a.m., regardless of how often he nursed in the night.
* He should be offered up to 20–25 minutes on the full breast, then up to 10–15 minutes on the second breast.
* Do not feed after 7:45 a.m. He can stay awake for up to two hours.

8 A.M.
* It is very important that you have a breakfast of cereal, toast and a drink no later than 8 a.m.

9 A.M.
* If your baby has not been settling well for his nap, offer him up to 5–10 minutes on the breast from which he last fed.
* Try to have a short rest when the baby is sleeping.

10 A.M.

* **Baby must be fully awake now, regardless of how long he slept.**
* He should be given up to 20–25 minutes from the breast he last fed on while you drink a glass of water and have a small snack.
* Express 2 oz. from the second breast, then offer him up to 10–20 minutes on the same breast.

11:45 A.M.

* He should be given the 2 oz. that you expressed to ensure that he does not wake hungry from his midday nap.
* It is very important that you have a good lunch and a rest before the next feeding.

2 P.M.

* **Baby should be awake and eating no later than 2 p.m., regardless of how long he has slept.**
* Give him up to 20–25 minutes from the breast he last nursed from while you drink a glass of water. Express 2 oz. from the second breast, and then offer up to 10–20 minutes on the same breast.

4 P.M.

* Baby will need a short nap according to the routine appropriate for his age.

5 P.M.

* **Baby should be fully awake and eating no later than 5 p.m.**
* Give up to 15–20 minutes from both breasts.

6:15 P.M.

* Baby should be offered a top-up of expressed milk from the bottle. A baby less than 8 lbs. in weight will probably settle with 2–3 oz.; bigger babies may need 4–5 oz.

* Once your baby is settled, it is important that you have a good meal and a rest.

8 P.M.

* Express from both breasts.

10 P.M.

* It is important that you express from both breasts at this time, as the amount you get will be a good indicator of how much milk you are producing.

* Arrange for your partner or another family member to give the late feeding to the baby so you can have an early night.

10:30 P.M.

* Baby should be awake and eating no later than 10:30 p.m. He can be given a full feeding of either formula or expressed milk from a bottle. Refer to Chapter Three, Milk Feeding in the First Year, for details of the amounts to give.

In the Night

A baby who has had a full feeding from the bottle at 10:30 p.m. should feel satisfied until 2–2:30 a.m. He should then be offered 20–25 minutes from the first breast, then 10–15 minutes from the second. In order to avoid a second waking in the night at 5 a.m., it is very important that he nurses from both breasts.

······

If your baby ate well at 10:30 p.m. and wakes earlier than 2 a.m., the cause may not be hunger. The following are other reasons which may be causing him to wake earlier.

Kicking off the covers may be the cause of your baby waking earlier than 2 a.m. A baby less than six weeks who wakes thrashing around may still need to be fully swaddled. A baby more than six weeks may benefit from being half-swaddled under the arms in a thin cotton sheet. With all babies, it is important to ensure that the top sheet is tucked in well, down the sides and at the bottom of the crib.

The baby should be fully awake at the late feeding. With a baby who is waking before 2 a.m., it may be worthwhile keeping him awake longer, and offering him some more milk just before you settle him at around 11:15 p.m.

Day Four

* By day four, your breasts should be feeling fuller in the morning and the following alterations should be made to the plan:
* If your baby is sleeping well between 9 a.m. and 9:45 a.m., reduce the time on the breast at 9 a.m. to five minutes.
* The top-up at 11:45 a.m. can be reduced by 1 oz. if he is sleeping well at lunchtime or shows signs of not feeding well at the 2 p.m. feeding.
* The expressing at the 2 p.m. feeding should be dropped, which should mean that your breasts are fuller at 5 p.m.
* If you feel your breasts are fuller at 5 p.m., make sure he totally empties the first breast before putting him onto the second breast. If he has not emptied the second breast before his bath, he should be offered it again after the bath, and before he is given a top-up.

✳ The 8 p.m. expressing should be dropped and the 10 p.m. expressing brought forward to 9:30 p.m. It is important that both breasts are completely emptied at the 9:30 p.m. expressing.

Day Five

Dropping the 2 p.m. and 8 p.m. expressing on the fourth day should result in your breasts being very engorged on the morning of the fifth day; it is very important that the extra milk is totally emptied at the baby's first meal in the morning.

✳ At the 7 a.m. feeding, the baby should be offered up to 20–25 minutes on the fuller breast, then up to 10–15 minutes on the second breast, after you have expressed. The amount you express will depend upon the weight of your baby. It is important that you take just the right amount so that enough is left for your baby to get a full feeding. If you managed to express at least 4 oz. at the late feeding, you should manage to express the following amounts:

(a) Baby weighing 8–10 lbs.—express 4 oz.

(b) Baby weighing 10–12 lbs.—express 3 oz.

(c) Baby weighing more than 12 lbs.—express 2 oz.

Day Six

By the sixth day, your milk supply should have increased enough for you to drop all top-up feedings and follow the breast-feeding routines appropriate for your baby's age. It is very important that you also follow the guidelines for expressing as set in the routines. This will ensure that you will be able to satisfy your baby's increased appetite during his next growth spurt. I would also suggest that you continue with one bottle of either expressed or formula milk at the late feeding until your baby is introduced to solids at six months. This will allow the feeding to be given by your husband or partner, enabling you to get to bed after you have expressed, which, in turn, will make it easier for you to cope with the middle-of-the-night feeding.

Excessive Night Feeding

I have found that all babies, even demand-fed babies, are capable of sleeping one longer spell between feedings by the time they reach 4–6 weeks of age. Beatrice Hollyer and Lucy Smith, authors of the excellent book *Sleep: The Secret of Problem-free Nights*, describe this longer stretch of sleep as the "core night." They advise parents to take their cue from this longer stretch of sleeping, which they believe is the foundation of encouraging a baby to sleep right through the night.

I believe that by the end of the second week a baby who weighed 7 lbs. or more at birth should really only need one feeding in the night (between midnight and 6 a.m.). This is provided, of course, that he is eating well at all of his daytime feedings and gets a full feeding between 10 p.m. and 11 p.m. In my experience, regardless of whether he is breast- or bottle-fed, a baby who continues to nurse 2–3 times in the night will eventually begin to cut back on his daytime feedings. A vicious circle soon emerges, in which the baby ends up genuinely needing to eat in the night so that his daily nutritional needs can be met.

With bottle-fed babies, it is easier to avoid a pattern of excessive nighttime feeding by monitoring the amounts they are getting during the day. Calculate how much milk your baby needs each day for his weight. Then use the example chart in Chapter

Three, Milk Feeding in the First Year, to see how to structure feedings, so the biggest feedings are at the night times. This, as well as the core-night suggestions (later in this section), will prevent excessive night feeding for a formula-fed baby.

Excessive nighttime feeding is considered normal for breast-fed babies and is actually encouraged by many breast-feeding experts. Mothers are advised to have their baby sleep with them, so that he can feed on and off throughout the night. Much emphasis is placed on the fact that the hormone prolactin, which is necessary for making breast milk, is produced more at night. The theory is that mothers who nurse their babies more in the night than in the day are much more likely to sustain a good milk supply. This advice obviously works for some mothers, but breast-feeding statistics prove that it clearly doesn't for many others, as so many give up in the first month. As I've said, I believe that the exhaustion caused by so many nighttime feedings is one of the main reasons why so many mothers give up altogether.

In my experience from working with hundreds of breast-feeding mothers, I have found that a good stretch of sleep in the night results in the breasts producing more milk. A full and satisfying feeding in the middle of the night will ensure that the baby settles back to sleep quickly until the morning.

The following list gives the main causes of excessive nighttime feeding and how to avoid it:

* A premature baby or a very tiny baby would need to feed more often than every three hours, and medical advice should be sought on how best to deal with these special circumstances.
* If he nurses well at every feeding (a baby more than 8 lbs. should always be offered the second breast) and is

sleeping well at all the other sleep times, he may not be getting enough from the late feeding.

✳ If a low milk supply at the last feeding is the problem, it can easily be solved by ensuring your baby takes a full feeding from a bottle of either formula or expressed milk.

✳ Many women are concerned that introducing a bottle too early may reduce the baby's desire to take the breast. All of my babies are offered one bottle a day as a matter of course, and I have never had one baby who had nipple confusion or refused the breast. An occasional bottle has the added advantage that the partner can give the last feeding and enable the mother to get to bed by 10 p.m.

✳ If after one week of giving a full feeding late in the evening, there is no improvement, and your baby is still waking several times a night, it is more likely that he has a problem with his sleeping than with his eating. I suggest that you continue to offer the bottle for a further week and refer to "Excessive Night Waking" in this chapter for more advice on the subject.

✳ Babies less than 8 lbs. who are changed to the second breast before reaching the fatty, rich hind milk in the first breast will be more likely to wake more than once in the night.

✳ If a baby weighs more than 8 lbs. at birth and is only to nurse from one breast at a feeding, then he may not be getting enough milk and should be offered the second breast at some or all of his feedings. If he has nursed for 20–25 minutes on the first breast then try to get him to take 5–10 minutes from the second. If he refuses, try waiting 15–20 minutes before offering it again.

The majority of the babies on my routines who are feeding only once in the night gradually push themselves right through to morning, dropping the middle-of-the-night feeding as soon as they are physically capable. However, occasionally I get a baby who reaches six weeks and continues to wake at 2 a.m. looking for milk. In my experience, allowing these babies to continue to eat at this time causes them to reduce the amount they take at 7 a.m., often cutting this feeding out altogether. When this happens, I use the core-night method as follows to ensure that when the baby is ready to reduce the number of feedings he is having over a 24-hour period, it is always the middle-of-the-night feeding that he drops first.

The Core Night

The core-night method has been used for many years by maternity nurses and parents who believe in routine. It works on the principle that once a baby sleeps for one longer spell in the night, he should never again be fed during those hours in the core night. If he wakes during those hours, he should be left for a few minutes to settle himself back to sleep. If he refuses to settle, then other methods apart from feeding should be used to settle him. Hollyer and Smith recommend patting, offering a pacifier or giving a sip of water. Attention should be kept to a minimum while reassuring the baby that you are there. They claim that following this approach will, within days, have your baby sleeping at least the hours of his first core night. It also teaches the baby the most important two sleep skills: how to go to sleep and how to go back to sleep after surfacing from a non-REM (rapid eye movement) sleep.

Read the following points carefully to make sure that your baby really is capable of going for a longer spell in the night:

✳ These methods should never be used with a very small baby or a baby who is not gaining weight. A doctor should always see a baby who is not gaining weight.

✳ The above methods should only be used if your baby is gaining weight steadily and if you are sure that his last feeding was substantial enough to help him sleep for the longer stretch in the night.

✳ The main sign that a baby is ready to cut down on a night feeding is a regular weight gain and reluctance to eat or tendency to eat less at 7 a.m.

✳ The aim of using any of the previous methods is gradually to increase the length of time your baby can go from his last feeding and not to eliminate the night feeding right away.

✳ The core-night method can be used if, over three or four nights, a baby has shown signs that he is capable of sleeping for a longer stretch.

✳ It can be used to reduce the number of times a demand-fed baby is fed in the night and to encourage a longer stretch between feedings or after his last daytime meal.

How Giving Water in the Night Can Cause Problems

I advise that a baby between 8 and 12 weeks who is gaining at least 6 oz. of weight each week, yet still waking around 2/3 a.m., may be waking out of habit rather than hunger. In these circumstances, I suggest offering a small drink of cool boiled water. It is important that this advice be followed only if your baby takes the water and then settles back to sleep quickly for a reasonable length of time.

It is pointless to keep offering water or to persist with the core method discussed previously, if your baby refuses to settle back to sleep quickly or wakes again after only 30–40 minutes. If you continue to offer water over several nights and your baby is not settling back to sleep quickly, you will actually be encouraging your baby to sleep badly in the night—which is the opposite of what you want to happen.

If you think your baby is waking out of habit and not hunger, it is fine to offer water or some other form of comfort as described in the core-night method for a few nights to encourage him to go back to sleep. However, a baby who gets into the habit of being awake for lengthy periods in the night will soon start to get overtired during the day and want to sleep. Too much sleep during the day can also cause excessive nighttime waking. Therefore, the core method should only be used if you see a definite improvement in your baby's sleep within a few nights.

In the long term, night feedings are easier to drop with a baby who eats quickly and settles back to sleep until the morning, than with a baby who is awake on and off and being offered water, the pacifier or cuddles to get back to sleep.

Sleepy Feeder

Sometimes a very sleepy baby may be inclined to keep dozing during feedings; but if he does not want to take the required amount, he will end up wanting to eat again in an hour or two. This is a good time to change his diaper, burp him and encourage him to finish eating. Making a little effort in the early days to keep your baby awake enough to drink the correct amount at each feeding and at the times given in the routine will in the long term be well worthwhile. Some babies will take half the feeding, have a stretch and kick for 10–15 minutes and then be happy to take the rest. The important thing that I have found with sleepy babies is not to force them to stay awake by talking too much or jiggling them about. By putting your baby on the play mat and leaving him for 10 minutes, you will probably find that he will get enough of a second wind to eat again. During the first months, allow up to 45–60 minutes for a feeding.

Obviously, if he does not eat well at a particular feeding and wakes early from his sleep, he must be fed. Do not attempt to stretch him to the next feeding, otherwise he will be so tired that the next feeding will also become another sleepy one. Top him up, treat the feeding like a night feeding and settle him back to sleep so that you can get him back on track for the evening.

Refusal of Milk

The amount of milk a six-month-old baby drinks will gradually begin to decrease as his intake of solid food increases. However, up to the age of nine months, a baby still needs a minimum of 18–20 oz. a day of breast or formula milk. This daily amount gradually reduces to a minimum of 12 oz. at one year of age. If your baby is losing interest or refusing some of his milk feeding, and taking less than the recommended amounts, careful attention should be given to the timing of solids and the type of food given.

The following guidelines will help you determine the cause of your baby refusing his milk feedings:

✳ Up to the age of six months, a baby should still be taking 4–5 full milk feedings morning and evening. A full milk feeding consists of 7–8 oz. or a feeding from both breasts. Babies less than six months who are weaned early on the advice of a pediatrician should not be given solids in the middle of their milk feeding. They will be more likely to refuse the remainder of their formula or the second breast. Give most of the milk feeding first, then the solids.

✳ A baby less than six months of age still needs a full milk feeding at 11 a.m., even if he is being weaned early on medical advice. Introducing breakfast too soon or offering too much solid food first thing in the morning can cause a baby to cut down too quickly or to refuse the 11 a.m. feeding.

✳ The 11 a.m. milk feeding should be reduced and eliminated between the ages of six and seven months.

✳ Giving lunchtime solids at 2 p.m. and evening solids at 5 p.m. is the reason many babies less than seven months cut down too quickly or refuse their 6 p.m. milk feeding. Until he is used to solids, it is better to give a baby his lunchtime solids at 11 a.m. and his evening solids after he has had a full milk feeding at 6 p.m.

✳ Giving hard-to-digest foods such as banana or avocado at the wrong time of the day can cause a baby to cut back on the next milk feeding. Until a baby reaches seven months, it is better to serve these types of foods after the 6 p.m. feeding, rather than during the day.

✳ Babies more than six months of age who begin to refuse milk are often being allowed too many snacks in between meals or too much juice. Try replacing juice with water and cutting out snacks in between meals.

✳ Between 9 and 12 months, some babies begin refusing the bedtime milk feeding, which is a sign that they are ready to drop the day's third milk feeding. If this happens, it is important to reduce the amount given at the 2:30 p.m. feeding, before eventually dropping it altogether.

Refusal of Solids

With babies of six months or older, the refusal of solids often occurs because they drink too much milk, especially if they are still feeding in the middle of the night. Every day I speak to parents of babies and toddlers who will barely touch solids, let alone eat three meals a day. In the majority of these cases, the babies are still being milk-fed on demand, some as often as two or three times in the night. While milk is still a very important food for babies at six months, failing to structure the time of milk feedings and the amounts given can seriously affect the introduction of solids. If your baby is refusing solids, the following guidelines will help you determine the cause.

* The recommended age to introduce solids is at six months. If your baby is six months and sleeping through the night from 10 p.m., this late evening feeding should gradually be reduced and eliminated.
* A baby is ready to be weaned when he shows signs that his appetite is no longer satisfied with 4–5 full milk feedings a day. A full milk feeding is either an 8-oz. bottle of formula or being nursed fully from both breasts. See Chapter Fifteen, Introducing Solid Food, for signs that your baby is ready for weaning.
* If your baby reaches 6 months and is having more than 4–5 full milk feedings a day, drinking too much milk may be cause his refusal of solids. It is important to cut back on his 11 a.m. milk feeding to encourage him to eat more solids at that time. By the end of 6 months, a baby's milk intake should be around 20 oz. a day, divided between three drinks a day and small amounts used in food. If your baby is still refusing solids at this

age, despite cutting down on his milk intake, it is important that you discuss the problem as soon as possible with your pediatrician.

Fussy Feeder

If milk feeding is structured properly during the early days of weaning, the majority of babies will happily eat most of the foods they are offered. By the time they reach nine months, babies are expected to be getting most of their nourishment from eating three solid meals a day. Parents are advised to offer their babies a wide variety of foods to ensure they receive all the nutrients they need. However, it is often around this time that many babies start to reject food they have previously enjoyed.

If your baby is between 9 and 12 months of age and suddenly starts to reject his food or becomes fussy and fretful at mealtimes, the following guidelines should help determine the cause:

✳ Parents often have unrealistic expectations of the amounts of food their baby should have, and serving too large portions can mislead them into thinking that their baby has a feeding problem. The following list, showing the amounts of food a baby aged between the ages of 9 and 12 months needs, will help you decide if your baby is eating enough solids.
  * 3–4 servings of carbohydrate, made up of cereal, whole-grain bread, pasta or potatoes. A serving is 1 slice of bread, 1 oz. of cereal, 2 tablespoonfuls of pasta, or a small baked potato.
  * 3–4 portions of fruit and vegetables, including raw

vegetables. A portion is 1 small apple, pear or banana, carrot, a couple of cauliflower or broccoli flo-
rets, or 2 tablespoons of chopped green beans.

* 1 portion of animal protein or 2 of vegetable protein. A portion is 1 oz. of poultry, meat or fish or 2
oz. of lentil and beans and peas.

✳ Self-feeding plays an important role in a baby's mental
and physical development as it encourages hand-eye
coordination and increases his sense of independence.
Between six and nine months of age, most babies will
start to pick up their food and try to feed themselves.
The whole business of feeding can become very messy,
and mealtimes take much longer. Restricting a baby's
natural desire to explore his food and feed himself will
only lead to frustration and, very often, refusal to be
spoon-fed. Introducing lots of finger food and allowing
him to eat part of his meal by himself, regardless of the
mess, will make him much more inclined to take the
remainder from you from a spoon.

✳ By the time a baby reaches nine months of age, he will
become more interested in the color, shape and texture
of his food. A baby who is still having all the different
foods mashed up together will quickly begin to get
bored with even his favorite foods and this is one of the
main reasons that babies lose interest in vegetables.

✳ Offering your baby a selection of vegetables of various
textures and colors at each meal in small amounts will
be more appealing to him than a large amount of just
one or two vegetables.

✳ Sweet puddings and ice cream desserts served on a regular basis are major causes of babies and toddlers refusing their main course. Even babies as young as nine

months can quickly discern that if they refuse the main course and fuss enough, they will more than likely be given the dessert. It is better to restrict desserts to special occasions and serve your baby fresh fruit, yogurt or cheese as a second course.

✳ If your baby rejects a particular food, it is important that he is offered it again a couple of weeks later. Babies' likes and dislikes regarding food fluctuate a good deal in the first year, and parents who fail to keep reintroducing food that is rejected usually find that their baby ends up eating a very restricted diet.

✳ Giving large amounts of juice or water before a meal can result in a baby not eating very well. Offer him drinks midway between meals, not an hour before. Also, at mealtimes encourage him to eat at least half of the solids before offering him a drink of water or well-diluted juice.

✳ The timing of meals also plays a big part in how well a baby eats. A baby who is having his breakfast solids later than 8 a.m. is unlikely to be very hungry for his lunch much before 1 p.m. Likewise, a baby who is having late-afternoon solids later than 5 p.m. may be too tired to eat well.

✳ Giving too many snacks in between meals, especially hard-to-digest foods such as bananas or cheese, can often take the edge off a baby's appetite. Try restricting snacks for a couple of days to see if his appetite improves at mealtimes.

If you are concerned that your baby is not consuming enough solids, it is advisable to seek advice from your pediatrician. Keeping a diary for a week that lists the times and amounts of all food and drinks consumed will help your doctor to determine the cause of your baby's eating problems.

· · · · · · · · · · ·

Common Sleeping Problems

Difficulties in Settling

If your baby is difficult to settle at nap times, it is essential that you pay particular attention to when you begin settling him and how long you spend trying to do it. The majority of babies have a hard time settling because of overtiredness or overstimulation. Once you are confident that you have your baby's feeding and sleeping on track, I strongly advise that you help your baby learn how to settle himself to sleep. Although it will be very difficult to listen to him cry, he will quickly learn how to go to sleep by himself. He should never be left for more than 5–10 minutes before being checked. From my experience in helping hundreds of parents with babies who have had serious sleeping problems, once a baby learns how to settle himself, he becomes happier and more relaxed. Once proper daytime sleep is established, nighttime sleep will also improve.

The following guidelines should help your baby learn how to settle himself:

✳ A baby who is allowed to fall asleep on the breast or bottle and is then put in the crib will be more likely to have disruptive nap times. When he comes into a light sleep 30–45 minutes after falling asleep, he will be less likely to settle himself back to sleep without your help. If your baby falls asleep while feeding, put him on the changing mat and rearrange his diaper. This should rouse him enough to go down in the crib somewhat awake.

✳ Overtiredness is a major cause of babies not settling and not sleeping well during the day. A baby less than three months who is allowed to stay awake for longer than two hours at a time may become so overtired that he fights sleep for a further two hours. After three months, the majority of babies, as they get older, will manage to stay awake slightly longer, sometimes up to 2½ hours at a time.

✳ Overhandling before sleep time is another major problem with young babies. Everyone wants just one little cuddle. Unfortunately, several little cuddles add up and can leave the baby fretful, overtired and difficult to settle. Your baby is not a toy. Do not feel guilty about restricting the handling in the early weeks, especially before sleep time.

✳ Overstimulation before sleep time is another major cause of babies not settling well. Babies less than six months should be allowed a quiet winding-down time of 20 minutes before being put down to sleep. With babies more than six months, avoid games and activities that cause them to get overexcited. With all babies, regardless of age, avoid excessive talking at put-down time. Talk quietly and calmly, using the same simple phrases: "Night-night, teddy. Night-night, dolly. Sweet dreams."

✳ The wrong sleep association can also cause long-term sleep problems. It is essential that a baby goes down in his crib awake and learns to settle himself. For a baby who has already learned the wrong sleep associations, this problem can rarely be solved without some amount of crying. Fortunately, the majority of babies, if they are allowed, will learn to settle themselves within a few days.

Assisting-to-Sleep Method

All babies differ in how much sleep they need. During the first month some will feed, stay awake for a short period, then settle easily and sleep well until the next feeding. However, if a baby gets into a pattern of sleeping well during the day and then not settling or sleeping well in the evening or at night or is erratic with daytime naps, there are usually several reasons. Once you have ruled out genuine hunger as a cause and are ensuring that your baby is well fed, I would advise that you try a solution that I call the "assisting-to-sleep method." The aim of this method is to get your baby used to sleeping at regular times during naps and in the evening, which will help him to sleep through the night as soon as he is physically able.

After genuine hunger and the wrong sleep associations, I find that too much daytime sleep is the most common reason why a baby does not settle in the evening or wakes frequently during the night. When this happens a vicious circle soon emerges in which the baby needs to sleep more during the day because he is not sleeping well at night. In my experience, the only way to reverse this with a small baby is to assist the baby to sleep. Once his sleep improves in the night, a baby becomes much easier to keep awake during the day, which in turn helps him to sleep better in the evening and at night.

The aim of the assisting-to-sleep method is to get your baby used to sleeping at regular times during naps and in the evening. Once your baby is used to sleeping at the same times for several days, you should find that you can settle him in his bed with the minimum of fuss.

For this method to work it is important that it is done consistently and by only one parent. During stage one of the method and for at least three days, do not attempt to put your baby in his bed at nap times or early evening. Instead, one parent should lie in a quiet room with him and cuddle him throughout the whole of the sleep time.

Ensure that he is held in the crook of your arm, rather than lying across your chest. If he is older than two months and is no longer swaddled, it may help to use your right hand to hold both his hands across his chest; in this way, he will not wave his arms around and risk getting upset. It is important that the same person is with him during the allocated sleep time and that you do not hand him back and forth or walk from room to room.

Once he is sleeping soundly for three days in a row at the recommended times, you should then progress onto the second stage and settle him in his bed. It is important to sit right next to his bed, so you can hold his hands across his chest and comfort him. On the fourth night, hold both his hands until he is asleep, and on the fifth night, hold only one of his hands across his chest until he is asleep. By the sixth night, you should find that you can put him down sleepy but awake in his bed, checking him every 2–3 minutes until he falls asleep. Do not settle him in his bed unless he has been sleeping soundly in your arms for at least three nights.

Some babies may take longer than three days to sleep consistently at the recommended times.

When he reaches stage two, at which he is settling within 10 minutes for several nights, you should try leaving him to self-settle, using the crying-down method described earlier in this chapter.

It will help your baby get used to being happy in his bed if you put him in it for short spells during the day—when he is fully awake—with a small book or toy to look at. For the lunchtime nap, if you prefer, you can take your baby out for a nap in his stroller. The important thing is to try to be consistent; the lunchtime nap should be in the stroller or in the house, but do not switch from one to the other midway through the nap.

Early-morning Waking

All babies and young children go into a light sleep between 5 a.m. and 6 a.m. Some will settle back to sleep for a further hour or so but many do not. I believe there are two things that determine whether a baby will become an earlier riser. One is the darkness of the room in which he sleeps. It would be an understatement to say I am obsessed with how dark the room should be, but I am totally convinced that it is the reason the majority of my babies quickly resettle themselves to sleep when they come into a light sleep at 5–6 a.m. Once the door is shut and the curtains drawn, it should be so dark that not even the faintest trace of toys or books can be seen. A glimpse of these things will be enough to fully waken a baby from a drowsy state and make him want to start the day.

How parents deal with early wakings during the first three months will also determine whether their baby will become a child who is an early riser. During the first few weeks, a baby who is waking and eating at 2–2:30 a.m. may wake around 6 a.m. and genuinely need to feed. However, it is essential to treat this feeding like a nighttime feeding. It should be done as quickly and quietly as possible with the use of only a small night-light and without talking or eye contact. The baby should then be settled back to sleep until 7–7:30 a.m. If possible, avoid changing the diaper as this usually wakes the baby too much.

Once the baby is sleeping and eating close to 4 a.m., waking at 6 a.m. is not usually related to hunger. This is the one and only time I would advise parents to help their baby return to sleep. At this stage, the most important thing is to get him back to sleep quickly, even if it means cuddling him and offering him a pacifier until 7 a.m. The following are guidelines that will help your baby to not become an early riser:

* Avoid using a night-light or leaving the door open once you have put him down to sleep. Research shows that chemicals in the brain work differently in the dark, preparing it for sleep. Even the smallest chink of light can be enough to awaken the baby fully from his light sleep.

* Kicking off the bedcovers can also cause babies less than six months to wake early. In my experience, all babies less than this age sleep better if tucked in securely. The sheet needs to be placed lengthways across the width of the crib to ensure that a minimum of 8 inches is tucked in at the far side and a minimum of 4 inches at the near side. I advise rolling up a small hand towel and pushing it down between the slats and the mattress on the near side to further secure the sheet.

* Babies who work their way up the crib and get out of the covers will benefit from being put in a lightweight 100 percent cotton sleeping bag and tucked in with a sheet as described above. Depending upon the weather, blankets may not be necessary.

* Once a baby starts to move around the crib and is capable of rolling, I advise that you remove the sheets and blankets and use only the sleeping bag. This will allow your baby to move around unrestricted, without the worry that he might get cold in the middle of the night.

It is important to choose a sleeping bag that is suitable for the time of year.

✳ Do not drop the late feeding until your baby has reached six months and has started solids. If he goes through a growth spurt before he starts solids, he can be offered extra milk at this time. This reduces the chances of waking early due to hunger.

✳ A baby who is more than six months old and has dropped the late feeding should be encouraged to stay awake until 7 p.m. If he is falling into a deep sleep before this time, he will be much more likely to wake before 7 a.m.

Excessive Night Waking

Until the mother's milk comes in, a newborn baby may wake and need to be fed several times a night. By the end of the first week, a baby who weighs more than 7 lbs. should manage to sleep for a stretch of 4 hours from the 10–11 p.m. feeding, provided he is getting the amount of milk he needs during the day. Smaller babies may still need to feed every three hours around the clock. In my experience, all babies who are healthy and well fed will, between 4 and 6 weeks of age, manage to sleep for one longer spell of 5–6 hours. By following my routines, this longer spell should happen in the night.

How long a baby will continue to wake for a feeding in the night depends very much on the individual baby. Some babies between six and eight weeks old sleep through after the late feeding; others reach this milestone between 10 and 12 weeks. Some take even longer. All babies will sleep through the night as soon as they are physically and mentally able, provided the daytime feeding and sleeping is being properly structured. The following list shows the main causes of excessive nighttime waking in healthy babies less than one year old:

* Sleeping too much during the day. Even very small babies need to be awake some of the time. The baby should be encouraged to stay awake for 1–1½ hours after daytime feedings. Between six and eight weeks, most babies are capable of staying awake for up to two hours.
* Not feeding enough during the day. If excessive night feeding is to be avoided, the baby needs to have six feedings between 7 a.m. and 11 p.m. To fit in this number of feedings, the day must start at 7 a.m.
* Not feeding enough at each feeding. In the early days most babies need a minimum of 25 minutes on the first breast and after this should be offered the second breast.
* Breast-fed babies will be more likely to wake several times a night if they do not get enough to eat at the late feeding; they may need a top-up.
* Babies less than six weeks have a very strong Moro reflex (see Chapter Four, Understanding Your Baby's Sleep) and can wake themselves several times a night by the sudden startle and jerk. In addition to being securely tucked in with an appropriate weight of sheet and blanket, these babies will benefit from being swaddled in a lightweight stretch-cotton sheet.
* Older babies often wake several times at night because they have kicked off their covers and are cold, or they may their legs may have been caught between the slats of the crib. A sleeping bag will help them avoid both problems.

❋ The baby has learned the wrong sleep associations. Between two and three months, his sleep cycle changes, and he will come into a light sleep several times at night. If the baby is used to being fed, rocked or given a pacifier to get to sleep, he will need the same assistance to resettle himself in the night.

❋ Babies older than six months are more likely to be woken several times a night by the nursery door left open or a nightlight left on.

❋ If the baby's milk feedings are reduced too quickly when solids are introduced, he will begin to wake in the night genuinely needing a milk feeding.

Sleepy Late Feeding Causes Excessive Night or Early-Morning Waking

In the early days, establishing a full feeding in the late evening will help enormously in getting your baby to sleep for his longer spell during the night. Earlier in the book, I advise that this feeding should be a quiet one in the nursery, so that the baby does not become overstimulated and then refuse to settle well. However, if your baby is so sleepy that he is not taking enough milk to get him to go one longer stretch in the night, then I suggest that you introduce a split feeding (see Chapter Six, Weeks One to Two). The success of the split feeding depends upon the baby being awake slightly longer and drinking more milk.

Some of the babies that I cared for were so sleepy in the early days that I would have to start waking them at 9:40/9:45 p.m. I would begin by switching on the light low, pulling back the covers, taking the baby's legs out of his sleep suit and then leaving him in his crib. I would allow 10 minutes, and if he was not starting to stir, I would then turn the light a little brighter.

Regardless of how asleep he was, I would take him out of the room by 10 p.m. at the latest. I would take him either to my bedroom or the sitting room, where I would have the lights and possibly the television switched on to create a more stimulating environment. I would then lay him on his play mat for a further 5–10 minutes if he was still not completely awake before I offered him the first bottle of his split feeding.

I would ensure that I made the formula slightly warmer than normal and would always prepare a fresh bottle for the second half of the split feeding, which I would give at 11:15 p.m. I would keep the baby as awake as possible between 10 and 11 p.m. With some babies, it would often take up to two weeks to establish this split feeding; but once it was established it really did help them take a bigger feeding and sleep longer in the night.

If you are breast-feeding, the same method can be used, only you offer one breast at 10 p.m., followed by the second breast at 11:15 p.m. Some babies may actually need both breasts at 10 p.m., and then be offered the second breast again at 11:15 p.m.—or perhaps a top-up of expressed milk if you feel your milk supply is low at this time.

If your baby is less than 12 weeks, very sleepy and not feeding well at the last feeding, it really is worth persevering with trying to establish a split feeding. For this to work at the late feeding, you would also have to be doing a split feeding at 5/6:15 p.m. If you drop the split feeding at this time, your baby will probably be taking a much bigger feeding after his bath, which would have the domino effect of reducing his appetite at the late feeding. In order for the late split feeding to work, you need to continue with the split feeding at 5/6:15 p.m.

If you have tried all of the suggestions and your baby is still not eating well and is waking early in the night, you may wish to try dropping the 10 p.m. feeding for several nights and seeing how long he goes naturally. Once your baby sleeps a longer spell for several nights in a row, you would then reintroduce the 10 p.m. feeding and, hopefully, the baby will continue to sleep this longer spell at the right time of night.

The majority of babies will continue to need at least one feeding in the twelve-hour night until weaning is well established at around seven months of age. Therefore, it really is worthwhile being consistent and persistent about establishing a 10 p.m. feeding.

Illness—The Effect on Sleep

The majority of my first babies manage to get through the first year without suffering the colds and coughs that seem to plague my second and third babies. By the time most first babies experience a cold, their sleep is so well established that waking in the night is very rare. With second and third babies, this is not the case as they usually catch their first cold at a much younger age from a brother or sister, and disrupted nights are inevitable. A baby less than three months old will usually need help to get through the night when he has a cold or is ill. A young baby with a cold can get very distressed, especially when he is trying to drink his milk, as he will not have learned to breathe through his mouth.

When a sick baby needs attention in the evening and during the night, it should be given calmly and quietly. A sick baby needs more rest than a healthy baby. Lots of visitors and activity in the area where the baby sleeps during the evening and in the night should be avoided. When I have had to care for a sick baby of more than six months who wakes several times at night, I find it less disruptive if I sleep in the same room as the baby. It enables me to attend to him quickly and I am less likely to interrupt the sleep of elder siblings by coming and going along the corridor.

Occasionally, I find that an older baby who has dropped nighttime feedings will, once he has recovered, continue to wake in the night looking for the same attention he received when he was unwell. For the first few nights I would check him and offer him some cool boiled water, but once I was convinced he was completely recovered, I would leave him time to settle himself. In my experience, parents who are not prepared to do this usually end up with a baby who develops a long-term sleep problem.

If your baby develops a cold or cough, regardless of how mild it appears, he should be seen by a doctor. All too often I hear from distressed parents of babies with serious chest infections that might have been avoided if a doctor had seen them earlier. Too many mothers delay taking their baby to a doctor, worried that they will be labeled as neurotic, but it is important that you discuss with your doctor any concerns you have about your baby's health, however small. If your baby is ill, it is essential that you follow your doctor's advice to the letter, especially on feeding.

The Lunchtime Nap

The lunchtime nap is a fundamental part of my CLB routines. Research shows that babies and young children benefit from a proper, structured nap in the middle of the day. As your baby grows and is more active, this nap will become his time to rest and recover from the morning's activities and will enable him to enjoy his afternoons with you and others.

However, I am well aware that in the early days a lunchtime

nap can sometimes go wrong. I understand the feelings of frustration when a baby wakes 30–45 minutes into the nap and, despite still being tired, refuses to settle back to sleep. Assuming that the wrong sleep associations have not been established, there are several things you can do to improve the lunchtime nap.

First, allow your baby a short time to settle himself back to sleep, provided you are confident that the waking is not due to genuine hunger. Normally, over a period of a week or so, if a baby is allowed 5–10 minutes of crying down, he will then start to settle himself back to sleep. Obviously, if you find that after 10 minutes your baby is not crying less, but is in fact crying harder, then he should be attended to. With a baby who is crying harder, I would offer half of the 2 p.m. feeding, treating it like a night feeding, so that the baby does not become over-stimulated by lots of talking or eye contact. I would then assume that the reason why the baby can't settle himself back to sleep is because his coming into a light sleep coincides with his starting to get hungry.

Hunger—Young Babies

To eliminate the possibility of hunger causing a disturbed lunchtime nap in very young babies, I would bring forward the morning feeding to 10/10:30 a.m., and then offer a top-up just before they go down for their nap. This way you can be confident about allowing them a short crying-down period, without worrying that they might be hungry.

If your baby continues to cry and fails to settle back to sleep, it is worth considering the amount of sleep he is getting at the morning nap.

Morning Nap—Younger Babies

If your baby is between one and six months old and sleeping for more than one hour in the morning, it could be that too much morning sleep is affecting his lunchtime nap. Depending upon how much sleep your baby is getting at the morning nap, I would try reducing it to between 45 and 60 minutes, maximum. Occasionally, with some babies more than three months old I have had to reduce the morning nap to only 30 minutes to ensure a two-hour nap at lunchtime.

If you find that you cannot push your baby as early as 9 a.m. for his morning nap, I suggest that you do a split morning nap for a short time in order to reduce his overall morning sleep time.

Allow him 15/20 minutes at the first part of the split nap, then a further 15/20 minutes at the second part of the split nap.

By offering your baby a top-up before his lunchtime nap, reducing his morning nap to between 30 and 40 minutes and allowing him a short spell of crying down when he does wake after only 45 minutes, he should start to sleep for a longer spell again.

Hunger—Older Babies

With a baby who is weaned, you can try offering a top-up of milk just before his lunchtime nap. If you find that he is taking quite a large top-up, it would be worth considering the amount of solids that you are giving and ensure that you are getting the right balance of protein, carbohydrates and vegetables.

By seven months, your baby should be eating three meals a day and solids should be well established. If you have weaned at six months, you will need to move through the guide quickly to build up the right amounts of food.

If your baby is more than nine months old and is not having

a good drink of water or well-diluted juice with his lunch, thirst can be a reason why he wakes early from his nap, especially during hot weather. It is, therefore, worth offering him a drink of water just before his lunchtime nap.

Once the possibility of hunger is ruled out, if your older baby's crying continues to escalate rather than diminish, then you should consider the amount of sleep he is getting in the morning.

Morning Nap—Older Babies

With babies more than six months old, try to ensure that the morning nap is not before 9:15/9:30 a.m. If you find your baby is sleeping longer than 45 minutes at this nap, this could be the reason why he is not sleeping long enough at lunchtime.

If your baby is between six and nine months old, reduce the morning nap gradually, cutting it back by 10 minutes every three or four days until it is down to 20–25 minutes. If your baby is between 9 and 12 months old, try reducing it to 10–15 minutes or cutting it out entirely. You may find that for a short time, if the baby is getting tired, you will have to make his lunch and nap a little earlier.

The top-up before the nap and the reduction in the morning sleep should see an improvement in the length of time he sleeps during the lunchtime nap within one or two weeks.

The Lunchtime Nap—Further Troubleshooting

If you find that your baby will not resettle back to sleep at the lunchtime nap, despite trying all of the previous suggestions, you will have to adjust his afternoon sleep routine, so that he does not become overtired at bedtime. The age of your baby will dictate how much sleep you give him later in the day.

A baby of 6–9 months may need a 30-minute nap after the 2:30 p.m. feeding and then a further short nap at around 4:30 p.m. This should stop him from getting overtired and irritable and will help you to get his routine back on track again by 5 p.m., so that he settles well at 7 p.m. Sometimes a baby doesn't sleep at 2:30 p.m., especially if more than nine months old, but will then fall asleep later, between 3–4 p.m., and then wake after 30–45 minutes. If this happens, you may find that you have to bring bedtime forward slightly.

The important thing to remember when adjusting the routines to make up for a shorter lunchtime nap is to try to follow the recommendations for the maximum amount of daily sleep for your baby's age. Also, try to make sure that your baby is up and awake by 5 p.m. if you want him to go down well at 7 p.m.

CHECKLIST

* Rule out hunger as the possible cause of waking by offering a top-up milk feeding just before the nap. If an older baby who is weaned is drinking more than a couple of ounces, it is possible he needs his solids to be increased. Some breast-fed babies, despite eating a good amount of solids, may need a top-up breast-feeding until past nine months of age.

* With an older baby, check to see if he is thirsty by offering him a drink of cool boiled water just before he goes down for his lunchtime nap.

* Correct any poor sleep associations, such as falling asleep on the breast or the bottle, and ensure that he goes down well fed in his bed. It might take some time to get your baby into good habits, so you will need to be patient.

* Eliminate all other reasons for waking, such as excessive noise or loose bedsheets. (Remember that the Moro reflex—see Chapter Four, Understanding Your Baby's Sleep—can be very strong in babies less than six months, so tucking them in securely is very important if they are not to wake themselves up.)

✳ Always allow your baby to wake naturally and, after the first few weeks, provided he is not screaming for food, allow him a short awake spell in his bed before you pick him up; in this way, he will not associate waking with being picked up.

If the lunchtime nap still continues to be a problem (and you feel your baby has gotten into the habit of waking when he comes into a light sleep), you have checked everything on the checklist and given any changes enough time to work, it may be worth trying the assisting-to-sleep method mentioned earlier in this chapter. This method can help babies to sleep at regular times, not just at night.

Crying Down During the Lunchtime Nap

In my books, I say that crying down can be used from a very young age with babies who fight sleep or are overtired. It is very important to understand the difference between crying down and sleep training so that your baby is not caused any distress and the problem you are struggling with is not made worse. The following is a brief summary of the method:

Crying down is appropriate when a baby who is well fed, tired and ready to sleep but fights sleep when put into the crib. He will usually cry on and off for 5–10 minutes before drifting off to sleep—although some very overtired babies may cry on and off for up to 20 minutes. Once asleep, these babies will then sleep for the full nap time or at night until the next feeding is due.

If your baby wakes after 30–45 minutes and then settles back within 10–20 minutes of fussing for a further 30–45 minutes, this could be classed as crying down. But if your baby wakes after 30–45 minutes, does not settle back to sleep and is left to cry for longer than the suggested time, then this is *not* crying down.

I do not recommend that babies be left to cry for lengthy periods. It causes distress and creates a habit of them crying the minute they wake or come into a light sleep. It is much better to get the baby up and allow him one or two short naps later in the afternoon, depending upon his age. In my experience, as long as parents establish the right sleep associations and learn how to adjust the afternoon nap so that their baby does not become overtired, their baby will eventually start to sleep longer during the lunchtime nap.

Sleep Associations

During the early months, many babies are happy to doze on and off in a car seat or baby carrier, which can be convenient as it allows parents more flexibility. Unfortunately, once a baby becomes bigger and more active, he is unlikely to continue to sleep well or for long enough in either one of these (and probably will have outgrown the baby carrier and bassinet by then). If this habit is established, it can be very difficult to get him to sleep in his crib during the day. The sleep in the car seat is unlikely to be satisfying, and as he gets older, he will most likely spend the time catnapping and become tired and irritable later on. As a result, he might not eat well at the late-afternoon snack or will fall asleep before he's had all of his bedtime milk. Night wakings due to hunger can then result, leaving all of you tired the next day and so the problem continues to get worse. You need to start putting him to sleep in his bed as early as possible. If you can't because of older children or other responsibilities, settle the baby in his stroller in a quieter part of the house so he has a better chance of sleeping undisturbed.

If poor sleep associations have taken root, you will need to focus on getting him to sleep during this nap period whatever it takes. This is known as the *assisting-to-sleep method* (see earlier in this section). Take him out in the stroller or the car and let him have the two hours he needs. I usually found that if I did this for a week or even 10 days, the baby's sleep cycle would adapt to it, and it was easier then to put him down in his crib with just a little bit of crying down.

Teething and Night Waking

In my experience, teething rarely bothers babies who enjoy a routine from a very early age and have established healthy sleeping habits. Out of the 300 babies I have helped care for, only a handful have been bothered by teething in the night. In these cases, it is usually when the molars come through and then only for a few nights. I have found that babies who wake in the night due to teething are more likely to have suffered from colic and have developed poor sleeping habits.

If your baby is teething and waking in the night but quickly settles back to sleep when given a cuddle or a pacifier, teething is probably not the real cause of his waking. A baby who is genuinely bothered by teething pain would be difficult to settle back to sleep. He would also show signs of discomfort during the day, not just at night. I advise you to check the section on excessive night waking and early-morning waking to eliminate other reasons for your baby waking.

If you are convinced that your baby's nighttime wakings are caused by severe teething pain, I suggest you seek advice from your doctor regarding the use of medicine. While genuine teething pain may cause a few disruptive nights, it should never last for several weeks. If your baby seems out of sorts, develops a fever and suffers from loss of appetite or diarrhea, a doctor should see him. Do not assume that these symptoms are just signs of teething. Very often I have found that what parents thought was teething turned out to be an ear or throat infection.

Golden Rules

Finally, here are some essential tips to avoid potential problems in the first year:

✳ In the early days I advise that babies can stay awake for **up to two hours**. This does not mean that they **should** be awake for two hours. If your baby settles to sleep well in the evening and after night feedings but can only stay awake for an hour or so at a time during the day, he is obviously a baby who needs more sleep. However, if your baby is not settling well in the evening or after feedings in the middle of the night and you have ruled out the possibility of hunger, then it would be worth gradually lengthening your baby's awake time by a couple of minutes every few days until he can stay awake happily for longer and sleep better during the night.

✳ I recommend that babies should be allowed **up to 25 minutes** on the first breast, not that they **must have** 25 minutes on the breast. Some babies are very efficient eaters and can take a full feeding in much less time. If your baby is gaining weight and settling to sleep well for daytime naps and at night, then you do not need to worry about how long he is on the breast. However, if your baby is unhappy between feedings and not settling well for naps, it's possible that he is not taking a full feeding. Try offering him the breast just before naps. If he then settles well, you can be fairly sure that hunger is the cause of him not settling. To remedy this I would advise seeking help from a lactation consultant to ensure that you are latching your baby onto the breast properly. Once you are confident about this, you should keep checking that he is actually swallowing and not just sucking when he is feeding. Very small babies who spend lots of time sucking instead of feeding can quickly become tired and pull off the breast before they have taken a full feeding.

✱ If your baby is crying in the early days, you should always assume he is hungry and feed him. Remember, when I talk about every three hours, the three hours are calculated from the **beginning** of one feeding to the **beginning** of the next feeding. This means there is really only a two-hour gap between feedings. I also say that, if a baby is genuinely hungry before the recommended feeding times, he should always be fed. However, if your baby is looking for a meal long before the recommended time for his age, you should also try to work out why. The cause with breast-fed babies is usually a low milk supply or the baby not taking enough while nursing. If your baby is formula-fed and not managing to go three hours between feedings, you should consult your pediatrician.

✳ Do not move on to the next routine until your baby shows signs that he is ready to stay awake longer and go longer between feedings. Depending upon your baby's individual needs, you may find that he is sometimes between two routines. This may result in following sleeping times from one routine and feeding times from the next, or vice versa, but this is fine.

✳ Remember, the aim of the routines is to establish healthy long-term sleeping and feeding habits. A baby will sleep through the night as soon as he is physically and mentally able. You should not try to push your baby through the night by restricting or reducing night feedings too quickly.

✳ To avoid early-morning waking, ensure that in the first few weeks when your baby wakes in the night, you feed him enough to satisfy him until close to 7 a.m. In addition, once he is sleeping to 5/6 a.m. you should not leave him for lengthy periods to see if he will settle back to sleep. A baby who gets into the habit of being awake for any length of time between 5 a.m. and 7 a.m. is much more likely to develop a long-term early-morning waking problem than a baby who is fed quickly and settled back to sleep.

✳ It is also important that you do not reduce the time your baby is awake at the late feeding until he is sleeping regularly until 7 a.m. If he reaches three months of age and is not sleeping until close to 7 a.m., it is worth splitting the late feeding and having him awake longer at that time. In my experience, the split feeding nearly always helps very young babies sleep longer into the night; with older babies who were waking at 5 a.m., it helps them to stay asleep until closer to 7 a.m. Refer to Chapter Six,

Weeks One and Two, for details on how to implement the split feeding, and allow at least a week to establish it. The key to the success of the split feeding is ensuring that you wake the baby no later than 9:45 p.m. and keep him fully awake for the recommended time.

✳ Babies more than six months old who have dropped the late feeding and start to wake between 5 and 6 a.m. but do not settle back to sleep within 10 to 15 minutes should be offered a breast or bottle, even if the cause is not hunger. In my experience feeding the baby is the quickest way to avoid long-term early-morning waking. At the age when solids are established, too much day-time sleep is usually the cause of early-morning waking. Trying to reduce daytime sleep with a baby who is waking early is very difficult, hence the reason for offering a feeding as, unlike offering a pacifier or cuddles, it allows the baby to settle himself back to sleep. Then, as the baby sleeps better between 5 a.m. and 7 a.m., gradually push the 9 a.m. nap on to 9:30 a.m. and reduce it to 30 minutes. This will then enable you to push the lunchtime nap on to 12:30 p.m. and will eliminate any late-afternoon nap. Once your baby's daytime sleep is reduced you will probably find that he will naturally start to remain asleep until closer to 7 a.m. and will drop the early-morning feeding. However, if he has been sleeping through to close to 7 a.m. for at least two weeks and you find that you are still feeding him between 5 a.m. and 6 a.m., you can start to reduce the amount of milk you give him. Once you reach a stage where he is settling back with only the smallest amount, you can then drop the feeding and allow him to settle himself back to sleep.

• Appendix •

. . . .

NIH: National Institute of Child Health and Human Development Advice to Reduce the Risk of Crib Death

✻ Sudden infant death syndrome (SIDS) is the sudden, unexplained death of an infant younger than one year old. Some people call SIDS "crib death" because many babies who die of SIDS are found in their cribs.

✻ SIDS is the leading cause of death in children between one month and one year old. Most SIDS deaths occur when babies are between two months and four months old. Although health-care professionals don't know what causes SIDS, they do know ways to reduce the risk. These methods include the following:

* Placing babies on their backs to sleep, even for short naps—"tummy time" is for when babies are awake and someone is watching
* Using a firm sleep surface, such as a crib mattress covered with a fitted sheet
* Keeping soft objects and loose bedding away from sleep area
* Making sure babies don't get too hot—keep the room at a comfortable temperature for an adult

Source: www.nlm.nih.gov/medlineplus/suddeninfantdeathsyndrome.html

• Useful Addresses •

Baby products

Baby Center
www.Babycenter.com

Baby Gizmo
www.Babygizmo.com

Baby Earth
www.babyearth.com

Gibble
www.giggle.com

Target
www.target.com

Blackout lining and blinds

Hunter Douglas
www.hunterdouglas.com

Health and nutrition

Academy of American Pediatrics
www.aap.org
www.healthychildren.org

American Academy of Family Physicians
www.aafp.org

Mayo Clinic
www.mayoclinic.org

Lactation consultants

International Lactation Consultant Association
www.ilca.org

United States Lactation Consultant Organization (USLCA)
www.uslca.org

New York Lactation Consultant Association (NYLCA)
www.nylca.org

The Pump Station (Los Angeles)
www.pumpstation.com

La Leche League International
www.llli.org

Product safety and reliability

Consumer Product Safety Commission
www.cpsc.gov

Consumer Reports
www.consumerreports.org

Travel safety

National Highway Traffic Safety Administration
www.nhtsa.gov

• Further Reading •

A Contented House with Twins by Gina Ford and Alice Beer (Vermilion, 2006)

Feeding Made Easy by Gina Ford (Vermilion, 2008)

From Crying Baby to Contented Baby by Gina Ford (Vermilion, 2010)

Gina Ford's Top Tips for Contented Babies and Toddlers by Gina Ford (Vermilion, 2006)

Potty Training in One Week by Gina Ford (Vermilion, 2003)

The Complete Sleep Guide for Contented Babies and Toddlers by Gina Ford (Vermilion, 2006)

The Contented Baby with Toddler Book by Gina Ford (Vermilion, 2009)

The Contented Baby's First Year by Gina Ford (Vermilion, 2007)

The Contented Child's Food Bible by Gina Ford (Vermilion, 2005)

The Contented Little Baby Book of Weaning by Gina Ford (Vermilion, 2006)

The Contented Toddler Years by Gina Ford (Vermilion, 2006)

The Gina Ford Baby and Toddler Cook Book by Gina Ford (Vermilion, 2005)

Caring for Your Baby and Young Child: Birth to Age 5 by Academy of American Pediatrics (Random House, 2009)

Your Baby and Child by Penelope Leach (Knopf Doubleday, 2010)

The Baby Book by William Sears, M.D. and Martha Sears, R.N. (Little, Brown, 2003)

The Nursing Mother's Companion by Kathleen Huggins, R.N., M.S. (Harvard Common Press, 2010)

Healthy Sleep Habits, Happy Child by Marc Weissbluth, M.D. (Random House, 1999)

Dr. Spock's Baby and Child Care: 9th Edition by Benjamin Spock, M.D. (Pocket Books, 2011)

Secrets of the Baby Whisperer by Tracy Hoag with Melinda Blau (Random House, 2002)

What to Expect the First Year by Heidi Murkoff with Sharon Mazel (Workman, 2008)

• Contented Baby Newsletter •

Would you like to learn more about the Contented Baby routines and Gina Ford's books? Why not visit Gina's official Web sites at www.contentedbaby.com and www.contentedtoddler. com and sign up to receive her free monthly newsletter, which is full of useful information, tips and advice as well as answers to questions about parenting issues and even a recipe or two.

You may also want to take the opportunity to become part of Gina's online community by joining one or both of the Web sites. As a member, you'll find there are a huge range of benefits as well as a wealth of information and advice. You'll receive a monthly members-only magazine with a personal message from Gina, along with a selection of the latest exclusive features on topical issues from our guest contributors and members. You'll be able to access more than 2,000 frequently asked questions about feeding, sleeping and development answered by Gina and her team. You'll also find many case histories not featured in the Contented Little Baby series of books and an extensive archive of fascinating articles on parenting and lifestyle issues from experts on nutrition, diet, child psychology and counseling as well as from journalists and writers.

You'll be able to link with other parents on the forums in which you can discuss any parenting concerns, and you will be able to get in touch with other mothers in your area who are following the Contented Baby routines. You can even find out what Gina thinks about common dilemmas in her "Gina Responds" column. What's more, you can benefit from online shopping recommendations and tips on family days out.

www.contentedbaby.com

www.contentedtoddler.com

www.contentedbaby.com/store-directory

. . . .

Contented Baby Consultation Service

Gina offers a one-to-one personal telephone consultation service for parents who wish for special help in establishing healthy feeding and sleeping habits as laid out in the Contented Baby and Toddler routine books. If you would like further details on how a personal consultation with Gina works, we would request that in the first instance you send a detailed feeding and sleeping diary for 48 hours, along with a concise summary of what you think your problem is, using the contact form on www.contentedbaby.com.

. . . . . .

• Acknowledgments •

The first edition of *The Contented Little Baby Book* was based on my experience of working with hundreds of families around the world. I would like to say a huge thank-you to you all for having so much trust and faith in my methods and for the constant feedback that you have given me over the years as your babies have been growing up.

Keith and Janetta Hodgson deserve a very special thank-you for their invaluable help in transforming my routines and feeding plans into an at-a-glance form, making it easier reading for parents.

My family and friends have continued to be a constant support of love and encouragement. A loving thank-you to William Alexander Ford, Jean and Andrew Fair, Ann Clough and Sheila Eskdale, and to dear friends Jane Revell, Yamini Franzini, Jane Waygood, Jo Amps and Carla Flodden Flint.

My agent Emma Todd has also continued to give me the most enormous support and guidance, as has my publisher Fiona MacIntyre, editors Imogen Fortes, Cindy Chan and Louise Coe, and the rest of the team at Random House. I owe them all a huge debt of gratitude for having such faith in my methods and encouraging my career as an author.

A very special thank-you to my personal editors Dawn Fozzard and Gill MacCaulay, who have not only helped me greatly with my books and Web site, but whose emotional support, encouragement and friendship are a constant comfort and inspiration to me.

I would also like to say a very big thank-you to the Contentedbaby.com team, editor Kate Brian, Yamini Franzini, Frances Howard Brown, Gail Shearer and Sophie Huthwaite, for all the wonderful support they have given me personally and for doing such a great job of taking care of my Web site. Also to Rory Jenkins of Embado.com, whose technical skills have helped create a wonderful supportive community online that reaches parents across five continents. Laura Simmons, one of the founding members of Contentedbaby.com, deserves a very special thank-you for all her hard work in ensuring that the routines within this book are clear and concise, plus for the amazing support she has given both the members of my Web site and me.

I would also like to thank all the American parents who have used my book over the last ten years, and for all the wonderful support, feedback and appreciation that they have given me.

And finally, a heartfelt thank-you to the team at New American Library/Penguin Group (USA): Kara Welsh, Claire Zion, Ellen Edwards, Elizabeth Bistrow; and everyone in the sales, marketing, and promotion departments who have worked to support the book.

Finally, I would also like to say thank-you to the thousands of parents who have taken the time to write to me since the first publication of this book, telling me of the experiences of using the CLB routines. Your constant feedback has been very important to me and your loving, supportive messages mean more to me than you will ever know. Special love and thanks to you all and to your contented babies.

· Index ·